SBA for MRCOG 1

Dr Richa Saxena

Preface

This book, "*SBAs for MRCOG-I*" is intended for the doctors who are planning to appear in MRCOG part 1 examination. The MRCOG examination is meant for those doctors (undergraduates as well as postgraduates) who wish to pursue their specialisation in obstetrics and gynaecology in the UK. This comprises of a two-part examination (part I and Part II MRCOG exam).

According to the latest RCOG modules, the exam format for the MRCOG part I exam now comprises of SBA (single best answers) rather than the EMQ (extended matching questions), which comprised the previous exam format. The MRCOG part I exam comprises of two papers, with each having 100 SBAs. Therefore, a total of 200 SBAs are asked in this exam. For more information regarding this, follow the following link: https://www.rcog.org.uk/en/careers-training/mrcog-exams/part-1-mrcog/format/

Single best answer type of exam format comprises of a question with typically 5 options as answer. The candidate has to choose one of the best options as an answer. SBA is different from MCQ by the fact that the 5 options may include two options, which may pose as correct for the question asked. However, the candidate is supposed to choose the option which would serve as the best answer.

This book, SBA for MRCOG 1 is a compilation of nearly 500 SBAs commonly asked in the part 1 MRCOG written examination, which helps in the evaluation of basic and clinical sciences relevant to the subject of obstetrics and gynaecology. Fundamental aspects of all the important subjects related to basic sciences in medicine have been covered in this book. This is inclusive of subjects such as anatomy, physiology, biochemistry and nutrition, pathology, microbiology and immunology, embryology, genetics, biophysics, epidemiology, endocrinology and pharmacology. There is also a separate chapter on "Obstetrics and Gynaecology". The questions have been covered in accordance with the latest curriculum and examination format as described by the RCOG. Two model test papers comprising of 100 SBAs each would help candidates through self-evaluation.

Extreme care has been taken to maintain the accuracy while writing this book. Nevertheless, constructive criticism would be greatly appreciated.

Please e-mail me your comments at the e-mail address: richa@drrichasaxena.com. Also, please feel free to visit my website www.drrichasaxena.com for obtaining information related to various other books written by me and to make use of the free resources available for the doctors. Free resource for MRCOG exams is also available on this website. Detailed explanation for the SBAs is beyond the scope of this book and has not been provided in the text. For detailed explanations related to these answers kindly refer to my book "Textbook for MRCOG-1 Basic sciences in obstetrics and gynaecology", which is available on www.amazon.com and www.flipkart.com

—Richa Saxena

(richa@drrichasaxena.com)

www.drrichasaxena.com

Contents

1

PRINCIPLES OF EPIDEMIOLOGY

Choose the Single Best Answer (SBA)

Q 1. Which of the following statement is true about evidence-based medicine?
A. Combines clinical expertise and external evidence
B. Does not involve health economic assessment
C. Is restricted to randomised placebo-controlled trials
D. Is used to cut down waiting lists
E. Tries to rely on subjective measurements of disease outcomes

Ans. A

Q 2. A surgical team presented their data demonstrating an increased rate of post-surgical wound infection following gastro-intestinal surgery compared with published standards from the Royal College of Surgeons. What is the most appropriate next step to be taken up by the team who is undertaking audit in this case?
A. Data analysis
B. Data collection
C. Identify standards
D. Implement change
E. Needs assessment

Ans. D

Q 3. A vascular team intends to compare their results for aortic aneurysm repair with national standards. What is the most

appropriate next step to be taken up by the team who is undertaking audit in this case?
A. Data collection
B. Identify standards
C. Implement change
D. Needs assessment
E. Re-audit

Ans. A

Q 4. An 82-year-old female who has dementia and is a resident in a nursing home is reviewed due to a vaginal discharge shown to be gonorrhoea. You suspect elder abuse and wish to contact the police. What is the most suitable form of consent, which should be obtained in this case?
A. Consent from carer
B. Consent from court of law
C. Consent from next of kin if possible
D. No consent required
E. Verbal consent required

Ans. D

Q 5. Which of the following statement regarding "consent in clinical practice" is correct?
A. Parents of a mentally handicapped individual can give consent for her sterilisation.
B. Parental consent is required for a girl of 14 to have termination of pregnancy.
C. Jehovah's Witness parents can refuse blood transfusion for their children.
D. A mother-to-be can refuse consent to Caesarean section, even if it means the child will die or sustain serious damage.
E. An intoxicated woman who gets into bed with a man is, in effect, giving consent for sexual intercourse.

Ans. D

Q 6. A surgical team assessing post-operative complications

following surgery for vaginal hysterectomy has retrospectively collected data over the last 5 years on 133 patients. What is the most appropriate next step for the team undertaking audit in this case?

A. Data analysis
B. Data collection
C. Identify standards
D. Implement change
E. Needs assessment

Ans. A

Q 7. Which of the following is true regarding the standard deviation?

A. SD = SEM/(square root of n)
B. The SD equals the SEM in non-parametric tests
C. The SD is a measure of observation variability
D. The SEM determines the accuracy of measurement of the observations
E. The standard deviation (SD) is equal to the standard error of the mean (SEM)

Ans. C

Q 8. Which of the following is true if a characteristic is normally distributed in a population?

A. The median will be less than the mean
B. The mean will be of lesser value than the mode
C. The numbers of individuals above and below the mean will be equal
D. This implies that most of the population comprises of normal individuals
E. 20% of individuals will be more than two standard deviations from the mean

Ans. C

Q 9. For the data series: 2, 1, 6, 4, 2, which of the following statements is true?

A. The mean is 6
B. The mean is always identical to the median
C. The median is 3
D. The mode is 4
E. The standard deviation is 2

Ans. E

Q 10. Which of the following is true regarding the standard deviation of a group?
A. Is the square of variance
B. Is a valid statistical parameter for observations that do not have a normal distribution
C. Is numerically equal to the standard error of the mean
D. Can be used for the calculation of Chi squared test
E. Is a measure of the scatter of observations about the mean

Ans. E

Q 11. Which of the following statements related to statistics is not correct?
A. In a normally distributed population, 95 percent of the values fall in the range of the mean plus or minus two standard deviation
B. Standard error and standard deviation are synonymous
C. The chi-squared test can be applied to nonparametric data
D. The statement "p is less than 0.01" means that there is less than 1 percent likelihood of an event having occurred by chance
E. Variance is equal to the square of the standard deviation

Ans. B

Q 12. In a trial of a new therapeutic agent, the required sample size varies with which of the following?
A. Experience of the investigator
B. Level of acceptance of failing to discover a true effect
C. Level of statistical significance required
D. Type of statistical test to be employed
E. None of the above

Ans. C

Q 13. A report of a clinical trial of a new post-operative analgesic states, "In a comparison between the new drug and a placebo, a higher proportion of patients taking the new drug obtained relief from pain (p < 0.05)". In consequence, which of the following statements is correct?
A. The trial was well designed
B. Amongst 100 patients treated with the drug five would be expected to have a placebo response
C. The result may have occurred by chance alone in less than one in 20 occasions
D. The probable error of the observations is +/- 5%
E. The result should be regarded as not reaching conventional levels of statistical significance

Ans. C

Q 14. A diagnostic test has a sensitivity of 90% and a specificity of 95%. Which of the following statements is likely to be true in this case?
A. 10% of positive tests are false positive
B. 5% of negative tests are false negative
C. Sensitivity is equal to true positives / (true positives + false negatives)
D. Sensitivity indicates the test will be negative in disease.
E. None of the above

Ans. C

Q 15. In a clinical trial of a new drug treatment for inflammatory bowel disease, the following results are obtained:

	Drug	Placebo
Improved	46 patients	34 patients
Not Improved	14 patients	26 patients

Which of the following statement is true concerning this data?
A. Data can be evaluated by computing a Chi-squared test

B. Data can be evaluated using a Student's t-test
C. If the statistical probability that the difference between drug and placebo is 0.1 then the drug can be introduced into clinical practice
D. Pearson's coefficient of linear correlation could be used to test significance
E. The superiority of the drug over placebo is so obvious that formal statistical testing is unnecessary

Ans. A

Q 16. Which of the following is not true concerning the use of a placebo in a clinical trial?
A. Is associated with no effects
B. Should be identical in appearance to the drug being studied
C. Placebo studies are undertaken in patients with cancer
D. Is pharmacologically inert
E. Is best administered by a person who is unaware of the drug's identity

Ans. A

Q 17. A random selection of 1,200 adults agrees to participate in a study of the possible effects of drug X. They are followed prospectively for a period of five years to see if there is an association between the incidence of cataract and the use of drug X. What type of study is this?
A. Case-control study
B. Cohort study
C. Cross-over study
D. Cross-sectional study
E. Randomised controlled clinical trial

Ans. B

Q 18. Which of the following is true when evaluating a report of a clinical trial?
A. Control and treatment groups must be equivalent in size
B. Even if randomisation is conducted properly, chance differences are inevitable

C. Adequate sample size commonly produces false positives and false negatives
D. Results are invalid if the trial is not of double-blind construction
E. Withdrawal of patients from a trial by the investigator does not cause any bias

Ans. B

Q 19. In a double-blind placebo control clinical trial, which of the following statements is correct?
A. Some of the patients are not treated
B. All the patients receive a placebo
C. The patients do not know which treatment they receive
D. Everybody receives both treatments
E. The clinician assessing the effects of the treatment knows which treatment the patient has been given

Ans. C

Q 20. Which of the following statements concerning statistical tests is true?
A. Wilcoxon's rank test needs equal sample sizes
B. Student's t-test is a non-parametric test
C. Correlation coefficients vary between −10 and +10
D. Sigma (σ) is the symbol-denoting coefficient of correlation
E. $y = a + bx$ is a regression equation

Ans. E

Q 21. Which of the following is not true regarding the occurrence of errors in clinical trials?
A. Errors are more common when big samples are used
B. Type I error is more likely to occur when multiple t-tests are used
C. Type I error is wrongly rejecting the null hypothesis
D. Type II error is accepting the null hypothesis when it is invalid
E. Type II error is reduced by the use of a confidence interval

Ans. A

Q 22. In comparing confidence intervals with P values, which of the following statements is correct?
A. 95% confidence intervals are equivalent to a P value of 0.95
B. As the sample size increases, the confidence interval will increase
C. Confidence intervals refer to the target population
D. The confidence interval is approximately equal to the standard deviation
E. The P value measures statistical significance of result

Ans. C

Q 23. Which of the following is true regarding 95% confidence interval?
A. Can only be used in parametric data
B. It is a test of the null hypothesis
C. If zero difference lies within the 95% when comparing two groups to a treatment, it indicates the treatment is very effective
D. Is not useful when comparing data with another population
E. It is calculated at ±1.96 times the standard error of the mean

Ans. E

Q 24. Which of the following is a standard method of reporting the results?
A. Mean, standard deviation, and 95% confidence intervals
B. Median, range, and interquartile ranges
C. Odds ratio and 95% confidence interval
D. Rate and 95% confidence interval
E. Risk difference

Ans. C

Q 25. Which of the following is not a continuous variable?
A. Blood pressure
B. Gender
C. Haemoglobin concentration
D. Height
E. Plasma glucose concentration

Ans. B

Q 26. Which of the following is true in significance testing?

A. A Type I error is to reject the alternative hypothesis when it should be accepted

B. A Type II error is to accept the alternative hypothesiswhen it should be rejected

C. The probability associated with a Type I error is the significance level

D. The significance level is always set to 5%

E. The significance level is determined at the end of a significance test

Ans. C

Q 27. Which of the following statements regarding statistical evaluation is not correct?

A. The arithmetic mean is the measure to be preferred in data, which are symmetrically distributed

B. The geometric mean is always less in value than the arithmetic mean

C. The median is also called the measure of central value

D. The standard deviation is a good indication of distribution about the mean

E. The value of the variable, which occurs with the least frequency, is the mode

Ans. E

Q 28. Which of the following statements regarding statistical terms is true?

A. In a positively skewed distribution, the mean always lies to the left of the mode

B. In distributions, which are markedly skewed, the arithmetic mean is a more appropriate measure than the geometric mean

C. In non-parametric data, the mode is usually different in value from the mean

D. All the above

E. None of the above

Ans. C

Q 29. A cohort study suggests a statistical link between drinking a specific local herbal tea and the development of oesophageal cancer. Which of the following would suggest that the link is causative?
A. An odds ratio of 8:1
B. The finding of similar results in a number of studies
C. The finding that increasing consumption is associated with an increased rate of disease
D. All the above
E. None of the above

Ans. D

Q 30. In statistics, which of the following statements is not correct?
A. The mode of a distribution is the most frequently occurring value
B. Wilcoxon's rank sum test is a non-parametric test
C. In any set of observations, half of the observations are greater than the median
D. The chi-square test compares the observed and expected frequencies of an event
E. Infant mortality rate is the number of infants dying during the first year per 10,000 live births.

Ans. E

2

ANATOMY AND EMBRYOLOGY

Choose the Single Best Answer (SBA)

Q 1. Regarding the lymphatic drainage of the anterior abdominal wall, which of the following is true?
A. The cutaneous lymph vessels above the umbilicus drain into the anterior axillary lymph nodes, while the vessels below this level drain into the superficial inguinal lymph nodes.
B. All lymphatic drainage occurs into the inguinal nodes.
C. The cutaneous lymph vessels above the umbilicus drain into the supraclavicular lymph nodes, while the vessels below this level drain into the deep inguinal lymph nodes.
D. All the above
E. None of the above

Ans. A

Q 2. Which of the following is true regarding the human rectum?
A. Drains lymph to the pre-aortic nodes.
B. Has mesentery in the posterior third.
C. Is covered anteriorly by peritoneum along its whole length.
D. Has a blood supply from the terminal branches of the superior mesenteric artery.
E. Has appendices epiploicae.

Ans. A

Q 3. Which of the following is not true regarding the boundaries of epiploic foramen?
A. Anteriorly it is formed by the free border of the lesser omentum.
B. Inferiorly by the peritoneum covering the duodenum.
C. Posteriorly by inferior vena cava.
D. Posteriorly by superior vena cava.
E. Superiorly by the caudate lobe of liver.

Ans. D

Q 4. Which of the following vessel is not a branch of the internal iliac artery?
A. Iliolumbar artery
B. Lateral sacral artery
C. Middle rectal artery
D. Obturator artery
E. Ovarian artery

Ans. E

Q 5. Which of the following is not true regarding the appendix?
A. It is located in the retrocaecal recess.
B. The longitudinal coat of the appendix is derived from the three bands of taeniae coli.
C. Is supplied by branches of the superior mesenteric artery.
D. It is typically less than 10 cm in length in the adult.
E. McBurney's point lies two-thirds laterally from a line from umbilicus to the anterior superior iliac spine.

Ans. E

Q 6. Which of the following structures does not pass through the female inguinal canal?
A. Iliohypogastric nerve
B. Ilioinguinal nerve
C. Interior epigastric artery
D. Round ligament
E. Spermatic cord

Ans. E

Q 7. Which of the following is true regarding the femoral nerve?
A. Has a branch which supplies the skin of the scrotum
B. Lies within the femoral sheath
C. Lies lateral to the femoral vein
D. May supply part of the foot
E. Does not have the same origin as the obturator nerve

Ans. C

Q 8. Which of the following is a branch of the femoral artery?
A. Peroneal artery
B. The ascending genicular artery
C. The deep epigastric artery
D. Medial circumflex iliac artery
E. Superficial circumflex iliac artery

Ans. E

Q 9. Which of the following is not true regarding the femoral canal?
A. It contains a superficial inguinal lymph node.
B. It contains the lymph node of Cloquet.
C. Has the inguinal ligament as its anterior border.
D. Has the lacunar ligament as its medial border.
E. Has the pectineal ligament as its posterior border.

Ans. A

Q 10. Which of the following is true regarding the femoral nerve?
A. It arises from the same nerve roots as the obturator nerve.
B. It supplies lateral side of the dorsum of foot.
C. It gives a branch to the scrotum.
D. It enters the femoral sheath.
E. Saphenous nerve arises from the anterior division of femoral nerve.

Ans. A

Q 11. Which of the following is true concerning the great (long) saphenous vein?
A. Ascends posterior to the medial malleolus
B. Passes through the femoral canal
C. Receives blood from the posterior tibial veins
D. Passes through the cribriform fascia
E. Receives the blood from deep external pudendal veins

Ans. D

Q 12. A 63-year-old man in the surgical ward is complaining of numbness over the anterior thigh and medial aspect of his right leg. He is unable to extend his right knee and the knee jerk is reduced. He had undergone a femoral aneurysm repair 3 days ago.
Which is the most probable nerve damaged in this case?
A. Femoral nerve
B. Saphenous nerve
C. Femoral branch of genitofemoral nerve
D. Genital branch of genitofemoral nerve
E. Sciatic nerve

Ans. A

Q 13. Please choose the most appropriate answer regarding the innervations of various muscles from the given list.
A. Triceps is supplied by radial nerve.
B. Gastrocnemius is supplied by tibial nerve.
C. Opponens pollicis is supplied by the median nerve
D. Deltoid muscle is supplied by axillary nerve.
E. All are correct.

Ans. E

Q 14. Which of the following regarding the vagina is correct?
A. The paramesonephric duct gives rise to both the uterus and the entire vagina.

B. Is 7–10 cm long.
C. The urogenital sinus gives rise to part of the vagina and the proximal part of the urethra.
D. Becomes canalised at 22 weeks of gestational age.
E. Vaginal fluid has a lower potassium concentration than plasma.

Ans. B

Q 15. From which of the following is the nerve supply to the vulva derived?
A. Genitofemoral nerve
B. Ilioinguinal nerve
C. Pudendal nerve
D. All the above
E. None of the above

Ans. D

Q 16. Which of the following is not true regarding the vagina?
A. Is covered anteriorly by peritoneum.
B. Is related anteriorly and posteriorly to the Wolffian (Gartner's) ducts.
C. It is made up of keratinized squamous epithelium.
D. The lateral vaginal walls are in contact with each other.
E. All the above.

Ans. E

Q 17. The change, which occurs in the vagina at puberty, includes which of the following?
A. An increase in the pH
B. Reduction in the number of DoÅNderlein's bacilli
C. Exfoliation of superficial cells with pyknotic nuclei
D. Reduction in the glycogen content of the epithelium
E. The appearance of glands in the epithelium

Ans. C

Q 18. Which of the following is true regarding the vagina?

A. Has venous drainage to the external iliac vein
B. Is covered with peritoneum in its upper anterior aspect
C. Is lined by squamous epithelium
D. Is supplied in part by the pudendal nerve
E. Has an anterior wall that is longer than the posterior wall

Ans. D

Q 19. Which of the following statements about the cervix is correct?
A. Nulliparous cervix is slit-shaped.
B. Peritoneum covers the upper part of the vagina posteriorly.
C. The isthmus is part of the cervix.
D. Cervix is lined by stratified squamous epithelium.
E. The squamocolumnar junction is found at the internal os.

Ans. B

Q 20. Which of the following statements is correct concerning the ischiorectal fossa?
A. It is separated from the perianal space by perianal fascia
B. The fossa is crossed transversely by the inferior haemorrhoidal veins
C. The levator ani muscle forms the floor of the fossa
D. The obturator internus muscle lies in its medial wall
E. The pudendal nerve lies within the fat of the fossa

Ans. B

Q 21. Which of the following is true concerning the ureter?
A. Has the genitofemoral nerve lies anterior to it
B. Is seen lying on the tips of the transverse processes of the thoracic vertebrae
C. It is surrounded by Waldeyer's sheath as it passes through the bladder wall
D. Lies anterior to the renal artery at the hilum of the kidney
E. Passes into the pelvis over the bifurcation of the internal iliac artery.

Ans. C

Q 22. Which of the following is true regarding the ureter?
A. The muscular layer of the ureter consists of longitudinal and circular layers throughout its whole length.
B. Has a squamous epithelium.
C. It is 10–15 cm in length.
D. The early splitting of the ureteric bud may result in partial or complete duplication of the ureter.
E. It is of endodermal origin.

Ans. D

Q 23. Which of the following pierce the urogenital diaphragm?
A. Obturator nerve
B. Rectum
C. Ureters
D. Urethra
E. Uterus

Ans. D

Q 24. Which of the following is not true regarding the urogenital diaphragm?
A. It is formed by the sphincter urethrae and deep transverse perineal muscles, which are enclosed between two fascial layers.
B. It is situated in the anterior part of the perineum.
C. Posteriorly the two layers of fascia fuse with the perineal body.
D. The closed space between the superficial and deep fascia is called the superficial perineal pouch.
E. The inferior layer of fascia is called the perineal membrane.

Ans. D

Q 25. Which of the following tissues is paired with the appropriate primary germ cell layer of origin?
A. Endometrium—mesoderm
B. Pineal gland—ectoderm
C. Tongue epithelium—mesoderm

D. All the above
E. None of the above

Ans. B

Q 26. Which of the following structures do not arise from the Wolffian ducts?
A. Epididymis
B. Epoöphoron
C. Gartner's duct
D. Paroöphoron
E. Round ligament

Ans. E

Q 27. Which of the following statement is correct regarding the development of genitourinary system?
A. Ova originate outside the developing gonad
B. Sertoli cells are derivatives of primordial germ cells
C. The external genitalia do not differentiate sexually before the 12th week of gestation
D. The Müllerian duct is an invagination of ectodermal tissue
E. Testosterone determines the development of male external genitalia

Ans. A

Q 28. At birth which of the following changes occur in the foetus?
A. Pulmonary vascular resistance decreases
B. The aortic pressure decreases
C. The left ventricular pressure decreases
D. The right atrial pressure increases
E. The right ventricular pressure increases

Ans. A

Q 29. In the foetal cardiovascular system, which of the following is not correct?

A. Cardiac pulsation is present by the 30th day after fertilisation
B. Oxygenated blood is transferred to the left atrium through the foramen ovale
C. The ductus arteriosus closes during the last 4 weeks of pregnancy
D. The heart arises from mesoderm
E. The heart is formed by fusion of endocardial tubes

Ans. C

Q 30. Which of the following circulatory changes occur at the time of birth?
A. A 20-fold increase in lung blood flow
B. A rise in right atrial pressure
C. Anatomical closure of the ductus arteriosus
D. Flap closure of the foramen ovale
E. Anatomical closure of the ductus venosus

Ans. D

3

PHYSIOLOGY AND ENDOCRINOLOGY

Choose the Single Best Answer (SBA)

Q 1. Lack of pulmonary surfactant is associated with which of the following?
A. Is unlikely in infants born after 30 weeks gestation
B. Can be diagnosed by examining the foetal amniotic fluid
C. Increases the effort required for expiration
D. Decreases the surface tension forces in the lungs
E. Leads to poor oxygenation of the blood before birth

Ans. B

Q 2. Which of the following statement regarding the neonatal development is correct?
A. Liver stores sufficient vitamin K for the first few months of life
B. Blood volume is closer to 750 than 250 ml
C. Blood glucose level does not fluctuates much in comparison to the foetal level
D. Gut usually lacks certain enzymes needed for digestion of milk
E. Peripheral vascular resistance is higher than that of the adult

Ans. E

Q 3. Which of the following statement is true regarding human chorionic gonadotropin?
A. Has a molecular weight of approximately 130,000
B. Has a similar molecular structure to LH secreted by the posterior pituitary
C. Stimulates the corpus luteum
D. Reaches a peak level at 16–20 weeks post-ovulation and conception
E. Is steroid in nature

Ans. C

Q 4. The corpus luteum of pregnancy does not produce which of the following?
A. 17 Alpha-hydroxyprogesterone
B. Human chorionic gonadotropin
C. Oestradiol
D. Progesterone
E. Relaxin

Ans. B

Q 5. Which of the following is not true concerning transfer of various substances across the placenta?
A. Amino acids are actively transported
B. Calcium is transferred by passive diffusion
C. Glucose is transferred by facilitated diffusion
D. Immunoglobulin IgG is transferred by endocytosis
E. Oxygen is transferred by flow-limited passive diffusion

Ans. B

Q 6. The liver is the principal site for the synthesis of which of the following?
A. Synthesis of plasma albumin
B. Synthesis of plasma globulins
C. Synthesis of vitamin B12
D. Synthesis of vitamin C
E. None of the above

Ans. A

Q 7. Which of the following statements regarding brown fat is correct?
A. Relatively more abundant in adults than in infants
B. Contains lesser amount of mitochondria than ordinary fat
C. Is less vascular than ordinary fat
D. Stimulated to generate more heat when its parasympathetic nerve

supply is stimulated

E. Is more important than shivering in neonatal thermoregulation

Ans. E

Q 8. Which of the following statement regarding cholesterol is not correct?

A. Can be absorbed from the gut by intestinal lymphatics following its incorporation into chylomicrons

B. Can be synthesized in the liver

C. In the diet comes mainly from vegetable sources

D. Is eliminated from the body mainly by excretion in the bile

E. Is a precursor of adrenal cortical hormones

Ans. C

Q 9. Which of the following is not correct regarding the symptoms of intestinal obstruction?

A. Constipation

B. Crampy pain due to intermittent vigorous peristalsis

C. Distension due to fluid and gas proximal to the obstruction

D. Hypotension

E. Vomiting which is more severe with low than with high bowel obstruction

Ans. E

Q 10. Auscultation of the heart can provide evidence of which of the following?

A. The direction of turbulent flow causing a murmur

B. Aortic stenosis, if there is a loud pre-systolic murmur in the aortic valve area

C. Mitral incompetence, if a diastolic murmur is heard in the axilla

D. Ventricular septal defect, if a loud diastolic murmur is heard

E. Mitral stenosis, if an early systolic murmur is heard

Ans. A

Q 11. Severe diarrhoea causes a decrease in all of the following

except?
A. Body potassium
B. Body sodium
C. Extracellular fluid volume
D. Total peripheral resistance
E. Blood pH

Ans. B

Q 12. Lack of pancreatic juice in the duodenum may lead to which of the following?
A. The presence of undigested meat fibres in the stools
B. An increase in the fat content of the faeces
C. Faeces with a low specific gravity
D. A reduced prothrombin level in blood
E. All the above

Ans. E

Q 13. Which of the following is not true regarding portal hypertension?
A. The total vascular resistance of the hepatic sinusoids is increased
B. Portal blood flow through the liver is increased
C. The volume of fluid in the peritoneal cavity increases
D. A porto-caval shunt (anastomosis between portal vein and inferior vena cava) can decrease the tendency to bleed into the alimentary tract
E. A porto-caval shunt increases the risk of coma after bleeding into the alimentary tract

Ans. B

Q 14. Which of the following is not correct regarding absorption of glucose by intestinal mucosal cells?
A. Relies on a carrier mechanism in the cell membrane
B. Is blocked by the same agents that block renal reabsorption of glucose
C. Is impaired by blockade of active sodium transport in the cells
D. Involves the same carriers that are used for the absorption of

galactose

E. Takes place mainly in the ileum

Ans. E

Q 15. Which of the following statements is not correct regarding saltatory conduction of the nerve fibres?
A. Occurs only in myelinated fibres
B. Does not depend on depolarization of the nerve membrane
C. Has a slower velocity in cold than in warm conditions
D. Transmits impulses with a velocity proportional to fibre diameter
E. None of the above

Ans. B

Q 16. Changes in maternal physiology during pregnancy include which of the following?
A. Increased nitrogen retention
B. Mean arterial pressure of around 20 mmHg
C. Increased arterial PCO_2
D. Increased tone in the urinary tract
E. Increased renal threshold for glucose

Ans. D

Q 17. Which of the following hormone acts on cartilage and liver to release IGF-1?
A. Growth hormone
B. Prolactin
C. Somatostatin
D. TSH
E. ACTH

Ans. A

Q 18. In males, which of the following hormone facilitates the generation of spermatozoa?
A. GnRH
B. Somatostatin

C. Dopamine
D. LH
E. FSH

Ans. E

Q 19. Which of the following is true regarding prolactin?
A. Release is inhibited by metoclopramide
B. Release is inhibited by thyrotropin-releasing hormone
C. Release is increased by suckling
D. Has lower blood levels during normal sleeping hours
E. Is necessary for milk ejection

Ans. C

Q 20. Which of the following inhibits prolactin secretion?
A. Corticotropin-releasing factor
B. Dopamine
C. Gonadotropin releasing hormone (GnRH)
D. Growth hormone (GH)
E. Thyroid releasing hormone (TRH)

Ans. B

Q 21. Hyperprolactinaemia with hypogonadism is found in which of the following conditions?
A. Chromophobe adenoma of the pituitary
B. Addison's disease
C. Hyperthyroidism
D. Sheehan's syndrome
E. None of the above

Ans. A

Q 22. Possible consequences of hypothyroidism include which of the following?
A. A subnormal body core temperature
B. A tendency to fall asleep less frequently
C. Increased body hair (hirsutism)

D. Moist hands and feet
E. Prominent eyeballs

Ans. A

Q 23. Removal of the thyroid gland (without replacement therapy) leads to which of the following?
A. Reduced Blood TSH level
B. Reduced Blood cholesterol level
C. Increased Blood glucose level during an oral glucose tolerance test
D. Increased response time for tendon reflexes
E. Increased tremors of the fingers

Ans. D

Q 24. Which of the following occurs when secretory activity in the thyroid gland increases?
A. The gland takes up iodide from the blood at a slower rate
B. Its follicles enlarge and fill up with colloid
C. The follicular cells become more cuboidal
D. The follicular cells ingest colloid by endocytosis
E. The blood level of thyrotropin (TSH) increases

Ans. D

Q 25. Which of the following hormone is secreted within the posterior lobe of the human pituitary gland?
A. Oxytocin
B. Thyroid-stimulating hormone
C. Luteinising hormone
D. Adrenocorticotropin
E. Prolactin.

Ans. A

Q 26. Which of the following is true regarding oxytocin?
A. Is synthesised in the supraoptic nucleus of the hypothalamus
B. Causes milk ejection

C. Is a large polypeptide
D. Is released directly into the circulation from its site of production
E. Relaxes the uterus

Ans. B

Q 27. Which of the following is true regarding oxytocin?
A. Causes relaxation of myoepithelial cells in mammary glands
B. Has 10% of the antidiuretic activity of ADH (antidiuretic hormone)
C. Is synthesised in the posterior pituitary gland
D. Lowers the threshold for depolarisation of the uterine smooth muscle
E. The sensitivity of the uterus to oxytocin decreases as pregnancy progresses

Ans. D

Q 28. Type 1 insulin dependent diabetes mellitus is associated with which of the following?
A. About a 1:3 positive family history
B. Decreased islet cell antibodies with increasing time from diagnosis
C. An 80% concordance among identical twins
D. Low plasma glucagon levels
E. Insulin resistance

Ans. B

Q 29. Which of the following statement about testicular hormones is true?
A. Inhibin increases plasma follicle stimulating hormone levels
B. Testosterone in plasma is partly bound to albumin
C. Testosterone is excreted in urine as 17-ketosteroids
D. None of the above
E. All the above

Ans. B

Q 30. Which of the following is true concerning sex hormone binding globulin?
A. Has a lesser affinity than albumin for testosterone
B. Is the main binding protein for aldosterone
C. Is the main binding protein for progesterone
D. Levels are decreased during oestrogen therapy
E. Levels are increased in pregnancy

Ans. E

Q 31. Which of the following is not true regarding neutrophil granulocytes?
A. Are the most common leucocyte in normal blood
B. Contain proteolytic enzymes
C. Have a lifespan in the circulation of 3–4 weeks
D. Contain actin and myosin microfilaments
E. Are present in high concentration in pus

Ans. C

Q 32. Will the following factors lower the ESR?
A. Systemic lupus erythematosus
B. Female gender
C. Macrocytosis
D. Polycythaemia
E. Rheumatoid arthritis

Ans. D

Q 33. Prothrombin time is not increased in which of the following?
A. Aspirin therapy
B. Cirrhosis
C. Disseminated intravascular coagulation
D. Unfractionated heparin therapy
E. Warfarin therapy

Ans. A

Q 34. The conversion of fibrinogen to fibrin
A. Is affected by prothrombin
B. Involves the disruption of certain peptide linkages by a proteolytic enzyme
C. Is followed by reduced polymerisation of fibrin monomers
D. Is not inhibited by heparin
E. Is reversed by plasmin (fibrinolysin)

Ans. B

Q 35. A 15-year-old child is admitted to hospital with recent onset of widespread purpura (pin-head areas of haemorrhage into the skin). What is the most likely abnormality to be revealed by the laboratory investigations in this case?
A. Deficiency of vitamin K
B. Deficiency of factor VIII
C. Increased fibrinogen level
D. Platelet count 90 x 10^9 per litre
E. Deficiency of prothrombin

Ans. D

Q 36. Which of the following statement is true regarding blood eosinophils?
A. Have agranular cytoplasm
B. Are about a quarter of all leucocytes
C. Are relatively scarce in the mucosa of the respiratory, urinary and alimentary tracts
D. Release cytokines
E. Increase in number in viral infections

Ans. D

Q 37. Which of the following is correct regarding the deficiency of factor VIII (anti-haemophilic globulin)?
A. Increases the bleeding time
B. Is due to an abnormal gene on the Y chromosome

C. To 75 percent of its normal value results in excessive bleeding after tooth extraction
D. Causes small (petechial) haemorrhages into the skin to cause purpura
E. Affects the intrinsic pathway for blood coagulation

Ans. E

Q 38. Which of the following is not true regarding the respiratory centre?
A. Is in the medulla oblongata
B. Sends impulses to inspiratory muscles during quiet breathing
C. Sends impulses to expiratory muscles during quiet breathing
D. Is involved in the swallowing reflex
E. Is involved in the vomiting reflex

Ans. C

Q 39. Which of the following regarding the carotid bodies is not correct?
A. Are stretch receptors in the walls of the internal carotid arteries
B. Have the greatest flow rate/unit volume yet described in the body
C. Are influenced more by blood PO_2 than by its oxygen content
D. Generate more afferent impulses when blood H^+ ion concentration rises
E. The aortic bodies are mainly responsible for the increased ventilation in hypoxia

Ans. A

Q 40. Which of the following statement is correct regarding carbon dioxide?
A. Is carried as carboxyhaemoglobin on the haemoglobin molecule
B. Uptake by the blood increases its oxygen-binding power
C. Uptake by the blood leads to similar increases in H^+ and HCO_3^- ion concentrations
D. Stimulates ventilation when breathed at a concentration of 20 percent
E. Content is greater than oxygen content in arterial blood

Ans. E

Q 41. Oxyhaemoglobin dissociation curve shifted to the left in which of the following conditions?
A. Alkalosis
B. Hypoxia
C. Increased pCO_2
D. Increasing body temperature
E. Increasing concentration of 2,3-DPG

Ans. A

Q 42. Which of the following statement regarding the renal clearance of a substance is correct?
A. Is inversely related to its urinary concentration, U
B. Is indirectly related to the rate of urine formation, V
C. Is directly related to its plasma concentration, P
D. Is expressed in units of volume per unit time
E. Must fall in the presence of metabolic poisons

Ans. D

Q 43. As plasma glucose concentration rises above normal, glucose
A. Filtration decreases linearly
B. Transport maximum Tm increases linearly
C. Clearance increases linearly
D. Reabsorption increases and then levels off
E. Excretion increases and then decreases

Ans. D

Q 44. Hydrostatic pressure in renal glomerular capillaries
A. Is lower than pressure in efferent arterioles
B. Rises when afferent arterioles constrict
C. Is lower than in most capillaries at heart level
D. Falls by 10% when arterial pressure falls by 10%
E. Falls along the length of the capillary

Ans. E

Q 45. Which of the following is true concerning creatinine?
A. Has a plasma clearance rate equivalent to renal plasma flow
B. Is filtered out by the glomerulus
C. Is reabsorbed significantly by the proximal tubules
D. Plasma concentration does not change after protein ingestion
E. Plasma concentration increases during the first trimester of pregnancy

Ans. B

Q 46. In which of the regions of the nephron is the macula densa tissue situated?
A. Thick ascending limb
B. Thin descending limb
C. Distal convoluted tubule
D. Proximal straight tubule
E. Medullary collecting duct

Ans. C

Q 47. Which of the following is true regarding electrocardiogram (ECG) interpretation?
A. 0.16 seconds represents a normal QRS duration
B. 50 mm per second is the standard paper speed
C. Standard calibration implies that 0.1 mV is equivalent to a deflection of 1 mm
D. The PR interval is measured from the start of the p wave to the end of the QRS complex
E. The QT interval is measured from the start of the QRS complex to the start of the T wave

Ans. C

Q 48. Which of the following electrocardiogram (ECG) changes are associated with a suspected myocardial infarction?
A. In a subendocardial MI, ST elevation and T wave inversion

occurs in leads facing the infarcted area
B. Myocardial infarction cannot be diagnosed in the presence of right bundle branch block
C. Myocardial infarction causes "convex upwards" ST elevation
D. Right ventricular infarction can be diagnosed using a standard 12 lead ECG
E. True posterior left ventricular infarction is characterised by pathological Q waves, tall R waves and inverted T waves in V1 and V2

Ans. C

Q 49. Which of the following is true in the digestive system?
A. Fructose is mainly absorbed by simple diffusion
B. Glucose transport into the cell depends upon the active transport of sodium ions
C. Lactase activity increases during childhood
D. One molecule of sucrose forms two molecules of glucose
E. Polysaccharides are broken down mainly in the stomach

Ans. B

Q 50. Which of the following is true regarding gastrin?
A. Is predominantly produced by G cells located in the pancreas
B. Levels are decreased in atrophic gastritis (pernicious anaemia)
C. Stimulates gastric acid secretion in response to hunger
D. Stimulates insulin secretion particularly after a carbohydrate meal
E. Stimulates the growth of cells in the gastric mucosa

Ans. E

4

BIOCHEMISTRY AND NUTRITION

Choose the Single Best Answer (SBA)

Q 1. Which of the following is true regarding carbohydrate metabolism?
A. The principal carbohydrate used in body metabolism is galactose
B. Glycolysis is the process of glycogen formation
C. The pentose shunt is active in all cells of the body except red blood cells (RBCs)
D. The tricarboxylic acid (TCA) cycle is the common pathway for the oxidation of dietary carbohydrates, fats and proteins to CO_2 and H_2O
E. Acetoacetic acid and beta-hydroxybutyric acid are types of fat

Ans. D

Q 2. Which of the following is not true regarding the conversion of glucose to lactic acid?
A. Is an irreversible process in skeletal muscles
B. Occurs in a single enzymatic reaction
C. Is inhibited by high cellular concentrations of ATP
D. Is the only pathway for the synthesis of ATP in the red blood cells
E. Occurs in skeletal muscle when the availability of oxygen is limited

Ans. B

Q 3. Regarding the oxidation of pyruvate to carbon dioxide, which of the following is false?
A. Can occur under anaerobic conditions
B. Involves intermediates that are also involved in amino acid catabolism
C. Is impaired in thiamine deficiency states

D. Is regulated by the concentration of acetyl CoA in the cell
E. Occurs exclusively in mitochondria

Ans. A

Q 4. Which of the statement is correct regarding the various cell organelles?
A. Lysosomes contain enzymes capable of digesting cells and cellular material
B. Ribosomes "Read" the mRNA and build proteins
C. Golgi apparatus is involved in the modification of lipids and proteins with storage of material prior to export out of the cell
D. All the above
E. None of the above

Ans. D

Q 5. Which of the following is true regarding glycogen?
A. It is a branched polymer of glucose
B. It is mainly stored in the muscles
C. It is broken down by glucose-6-phosphatase
D. Its synthesis is stimulated by adrenaline
E. Levels in the blood stream are highest in the morning

Ans. A

Q 6. Which of the following is not true regarding fat metabolism?
A. Fat cannot be metabolised anaerobically
B. Brain can utilise fat as a source of fuel
C. Oxidation of fatty acids occurs in the mitochondria
D. Beta-oxidation of fatty acids is controlled by the supply of substrates
E. Liver can convert fatty acids into ketone bodies

Ans. B

Q 7. Which of the following is not true regarding arachidonic acid?

A. It is a second messenger
B. It is a fatty acid
C. It is a precursor of thromboxane
D. It is inhibited by aspirin
E. It is converted into prostaglandins

Ans. D

Q 8. Which of the following nutrients and the deficiency disorder related to it is correctly matched?
A. Ascorbic acid—night blindness
B. Cyanocobalamin—microcytic anaemia
C. Folates—sprue
D. Niacin—beriberi
E. Thiamine—pellagra

Ans. C

Q 9. Which of the following is not true regarding prostaglandins?
A. They are hydrophobic
B. They are synthesised from arachidonic acid
C. NSAIDs (non-steroidal anti-inflammatory drugs) act as their antagonists
D. Comprise of 18 carbon atoms
E. Bind to G-protein coupled receptors

Ans. D

Q 10. Which of the following enzymes act at the ratelimiting step of the glycolysis pathway?
A. Glucokinase
B. Hexokinase
C. Pyruvate dehydrogenase
D. Phosphofructokinase
E. Phosphoglucose isomerase

Ans. D

Q 11. Overall product of the glycolysis pathway is
A. Acetyl coenzyme A
B. Glucose molecules
C. Pyruvate molecules
D. 2 NADH + 2 ATP
E. 1 NADH + 1 ATP

Ans. C

Q 12. Net yield per glucose molecule undergoing glycolysis is:
A. One NADH molecule and one ATP molecule
B. Two NADH molecules and two ATP molecules
C. Two NADH molecules and one ATP molecule
D. One NADH molecule and two ATP molecules

Ans. B

Q 13. Which of the following is not an intermediate product of the citric acid cycle?
A. Alpha-ketoglutarate
B. Acetyl coenzyme A
C. Citrate
D. Oxaloacetate
E. Succinyl coenzyme A

Ans. B

Q 14. Which of the following laboratory technique is used for detecting DNA sequences?
A. Eastern blotting
B. Western blotting
C. Southern blotting
D. Western blotting
E. Northwestern blotting

Ans. C

Q 15. Which of the following best describes the function of low-density lipoproteins?

A. Transportation of cholesterol from the body's tissues to the liver
B. Transportation of cholesterol from the liver to the tissues around the body
C. Transportation of chylomicrons from liver to the tissues around the body
D. Transportation of triglycerides from the liver to other tissues around the body for storage
E. Transportation of triglycerides from the intestine to other tissues for storage

Ans. B

Q 16. Which of the following is correct regarding vitamin C?
A. Is found only in animal foodstuffs
B. Is not destroyed by heating
C. There are normally large stores in the pancreas
D. Unimpaired wound healing is one of the characteristic features of severe vitamin C deficiency
E. Excess vitamin C can lead to the formation of oxalate stones in the urinary tract

Ans. E

Q 17. Which of the following is not true regarding metabolism?
A. The metabolic rate is the amount of energy liberated per unit of time
B. Anabolism is defined as the formation of substances, which can store the energy
C. Basal metabolic rate (BMR) is defined as the metabolic rate determined at rest in a room at 12–14 hours after the last meal
D. The BMR of a man is about 500 kcal per day
E. The metabolic rate is increased after consumption of a meal that is rich in protein

Ans. D

Q 18. Which of the following is true regarding metabolism?
A. Oxidation is the combination of a substance with oxygen, or loss of hydrogen or an electron

B. Co-enzyme A is a high-energy compound, which is formed from adenine, ribose, pantothenic acid and thioethanolamine
C. A calorie is defined as the amount of heat energy needed to raise the temperature of 1 g of water by 1°, from 15°C to 16°C.
D. All the above
E. None of the above

Ans. D

Q 19. Which of the following statement regarding vitamin B is not correct?
A. Vitamin B1 (thiamine) deficiency leads to impaired collagen formation
B. Vitamin B1 (thiamine) stores in the body are adequate for up to 9 months
C. Vitamin B2 (riboflavin) concentration is higher in the foetus than in the mother
D. Vitamin B6 (pyridoxine) requirement in pregnancy is 2.5 mg/day
E. Niacin is synthesised in the body from tryptophan

Ans. B

Q 20. Which of the following is not true concerning nitric oxide (NO)?
A. Effects of nitric oxide are mediated through cGMP as the second messenger
B. It has a long half-life
C. Is synthesised in the endothelium
D. It produces relaxation of the smooth muscles
E. Its production is increased in normal pregnancy

Ans. B

Q 21. Which of the following is not true regarding phenylketonuria?
A. It is an autosomal recessive disorder
B. It is associated with defect in tyrosine metabolism
C. Screening for phenylketonuria is done using Guthrie's test in newborns

D. Screening for phenylketonuria is done using Kleihauer-Betke test in newborns
E. Treatment strategy involves life-long intake of diet low in phenylalanine

Ans. D

Q 22. Which of the following is not true regarding steroidogenesis?
A. Cholesterol is the precursor of all the steroids
B. Corticosterone is converted into aldosterone
C. Progesterone is the precursor of pregnenolone
D. Pregnenolone is formed in the cellular mitochondria
E. Testosterone may be converted to either dihydrotestosterone or oestradiol

Ans. C

Q 23. Which of the following is not true regarding prostaglandins?
A. They are synthesised from arachidonic acid
B. Are antagonised by nonsteroidal anti-inflammatory drugs
C. All prostaglandins consist of 20 carbon atoms, arranged in form of 5 rings
D. Prostaglandins are hydrophilic in nature
E. They bind to G-protein coupled receptors

Ans. D

Q 24. An iron overload is not seen in which of the following conditions?
A. Thalassaemia major
B. Polycythaemia rubra vera
C. Myelodysplasia
D. Haemochromatosis
E. None of the above

Ans. B

Q 25. Which of the following are true regarding protein metabolism?
A. Proteins contain about 16% nitrogen
B. Chains containing greater than 100 amino acid residues are called proteins
C. Proteins yield 4 kilocalories per gram absorbed
D. All the above
E. None of the above

Ans. D

Q 26. What is not correct regarding enzymes?
A. Are proteins
B. Heating usually results in a complete loss of enzyme activity
C. A change in pH has no effect on the activity of an enzyme
D. Are present in all cell organelles
E. Organic solvents will usually destroy an enzyme's activity

Ans. C

Q 27. Which of the following is not true regarding methionine?
A. Cannot be converted to cystine by the foetal liver
B. Can cross the placenta
C. Is a sulphur-containing amino acid
D. Is an essential amino acid
E. Is reabsorbed in the proximal convoluted tubule in the kidneys

Ans. A

Q 28. Which of the following is true concerning 1,25-(OH)$_2$ D3 (vitamin D)?
A. Facilitates calcium and phosphate reabsorption from bone
B. Stimulates the absorption of calcium and phosphate from the gut
C. Stimulates the excretion of calcium and phosphate into renal tubules
D. Levels are low during lactation
E. Is less active than 24,25-(OH)$_2$ vitamin D

Ans. B

Q 29. Which of the following is true regarding tetrahydrofolic acid?
A. Catalyses the conversion of glucose to glucose-6-phosphate
B. Activity is not inhibited by methotrexate
C. Is a coenzyme in amino acid synthesis
D. Is a precursor of folic acid
E. Is involved in purine synthesis

Ans. E

Q 30. Which of the following statement about vitamins is correct?
A. Vitamin K is water-soluble
B. Vitamin D is normally absorbed in cases of obstructive jaundice
C. Vitamin A is a water-soluble vitamin
D. Vitamins supply the body with energy
E. Vitamin D is bound to a transport protein in the circulation

Ans. E

5

PATHOLOGY

Choose the Single Best Answer (SBA)

Q 1. Which of the following is not true regarding polymerase chain reaction?
A. DNA or RNA can be used as the template
B. Helps in diagnosis of infection
C. In diagnostic PCR, the exact sequence at both ends of the target region must be known
D. Polymorphisms in the viral genome may result in amplification failure
E. Takes several days to complete

Ans. E

Q 2. Chemical mediators concerned in production of an inflammatory response include which of the following?
A. Globulin permeability factor
B. Bradykinin
C. 5-Hydroxytryptamine
D. All the above
E. None of the above

Ans. D

Q 3. Which of the following is true regarding amyloidosis?
A. Is a type of coagulative necrosis
B. Granulation tissue is a feature of amyloidosis
C. The amyloid deposits lie around blood vessels
D. Renal failure may be the presenting complaint
E. Rarely affects the liver

Ans. C

Q 4. Which of the following is true regarding inflammation?
A. Following trauma, there may be initial vasodilatation followed by vasoconstriction
B. A cell-free plasmatic zone adjacent to the endothelium of venules is only seen in normal cells
C. The margination of white cells phenomenon is very characteristic of chronic inflammation
D. Pyaemia is an essential feature of abscess formation
E. Kinins cause relaxation of the smooth cells

Ans. B

Q 5. Which of the following statement regarding berry aneurysm is correct?
A. Are associated with diabetes mellitus
B. Are rarely associated with polycystic renal disease
C. Most often found in the circle of Willis
D. Result from abnormalities in the intimal wall of the arteries
E. Result from atheroma

Ans. C

Q 6. Which of the following is not a predisposing factor for atherosclerosis?
A. Cigarette smoking
B. Diabetes mellitus
C. Hormone replacement therapy
D. Hypertriglyceridemia
E. Systemic arterial hypertension

Ans. C

Q 7. Which of the following pathogens is commonly isolated from intra-abdominal pus?
A. *Actinomyces*
B. *Bacillus*
C. *Clostridia*
D. None of the above

E. All the above

Ans. C

Q 8. Which of the following tissues is not capable of cellular regeneration?
A. Bone marrow
B. Epidermis
C. Liver
D. Myocardium
E. skin

Ans. D

Q 9. Which of the following elicits a febrile response?
A. Corticosteroids
B. Interleukin
C. C reactive protein
D. All the above
E. None of the above

Ans. B

Q 10. Rigors are characteristic feature of which of the following?
A. Acute cholecystitis
B. Acute pancreatitis
C. Acute pyelonephritis
D. Hodgkin's disease
E. Ureteric calculi

Ans. C

Q 11. Wound healing by secondary intention takes place in which of the following circumstances?
A. When the wound becomes infected
B. When the wound does not break apart
C. When the wound edges are brought together
D. When there is irreparable skin loss
E. All the above

Ans. A

Q 12. Which of the following regarding the pathogenesis of thrombosis is correct?
A. Contact with subendothelial collagen causes platelet aggregation
B. Prostacyclin induces platelet aggregation
C. Thrombin inhibits platelet aggregation
D. All the above
E. None of the above

Ans. A

Q 13. Which of the following disease is not associated with HLA-B8?
A. Graves' disease
B. Insulin-dependent diabetes mellitus
C. Multiple sclerosis
D. Myasthenia gravis
E. Sjogren's syndrome

Ans. C

Q 14. Which of the following is true regarding acute tubular necrosis?
A. Shock is a cause
B. The blood urea nitrogen/creatinine ratio is greater than 20
C. The urinary sodium is less than 20 mmol/L
D. Urine osmolality is greater than 500 milliosmoles/L
E. Urine specific gravity is greater than 1.010

Ans. A

Q 15. Which of the following is cause of generalized lymphadenopathy (LAP)?
A. HIV seroconversion illness
B. Q fever
C. Syphilis
D. *Toxoplasma gondii*

E. All the above

Ans. E

Q 16. Which obstetric complication has an increased prevalence in women with bicornuate uterus?
A. Breech presentation
B. Postpartum haemorrhage
C. Placenta accreta
D. Placenta praevia
E. Spontaneous miscarriage

Ans. A

Q 17. Within what timeframe from injury do macrophages replace neutrophils in case of cutaneous wound healing?
A. 2–3 hours
B. 6–12 hours
C. 18–24 hours
D. 48–96 hours
E. 8–10 days

Ans. D

Q 18. Which of the following tumour is hormone dependent?
A. Malignant melanoma
B. Adenocarcinoma of the prostate
C. Adenocarcinoma of the pancreas
D. None of the above
E. All the above

Ans. B

Q 19. Which of the following is true regarding sarcomas?
A. They are slow growing tumours
B. Include gastrointestinal stromal tumours
C. Rarely metastasise to lungs
D. Originates from embryonic ectoderm
E. Respond poorly to chemotherapy

Ans. B

Q 20. Which of the following statement is true regarding cell necrosis?
A. Caseous necrosis can occur in presence of *mycobacterium tuberculosis*
B. Is a natural sequelae of the cell cycle
C. Is not associated with the release of inflammatory mediators
D. Is reversible
E. Does not involve any changes in the nucleus

Ans. A

Q 21. Apoptosis is characterized by which of the following?
A. Cell swelling
B. Karyorrhexis
C. Release of inflammatory mediators
D. None of the above
E. All the above

Ans. B

Q 22. Which of the following is true regarding hyperplasia?
A. It can be reversible
B. It occurs in the adrenal cortex in the sufferers of Cushing's syndrome
C. It occurs in the uterus during pregnancy
D. All the above
E. None of the above

Ans. D

Q 23. Which of the following paraneoplastic syndromes is correctly paired with a recognized causal malignancy?
A. Acanthosis nigricans and bowel cancer
B. Carcinoid and fibrosarcoma
C. Cushing's syndrome and small cell carcinoma
D. Dermatomyositis and renal cancer

E. Syndrome of inappropriate ADH secretion and testicular cancer

Ans. C

Q 24. Which of the following statement is not correct regarding pheochromocytomas?
A. High serum levels of metanephrine are diagnostic
B. They are corticosteroid-producing tumours
C. Commonly develop in chromaffin cells of renal medulla
D. Surgical resection is the treatment of choice
E. May present with severe hypertension and palpitations

Ans. B

Q 25. What is the genotype in a case of complete molar pregnancy?
A. 45 XO
B. 46XX
C. 46 XY
D. 46XXX
E. 69XXY

Ans. B

Q 26. Which of the following is not correct regarding choriocarcinoma?
A. It is a malignant condition
B. Is more common in women above the age of 40 years
C. Can follow a normal pregnancy
D. Can commonly metastasise to the brain
E. Syncytiotrophoblasts are filled with eosinophilic material

Ans. D

Q 27. Which of the following statement is correct regarding the congenital absence of the uterus?
A. Has an incidence of 1:1,000 births
B. Has a chromosomal pattern of 45 XO
C. Hirsutism is commonly observed

D. Is also known as Mayer-Rokitansky-Kuster-Hauser syndrome
E. The ovaries are commonly affected

Ans. D

Q 28. Which of the following diseases is not associated with HLA-B8?
A. Graves' disease
B. Ankylosing spondylitis
C. Insulin-dependent diabetes mellitus
D. Myasthenia gravis
E. Sjogren's syndrome

Ans. B

Q 29. Which of the following is correct concerning shock?
A. There is metabolic alkalosis
B. Hypoxia may not be present in some cases
C. Capillary permeability is reduced
D. Hypokalaemia occurs
E. There may be coagulopathy

Ans. E

Q 30. In the presence of inflammation, which of the following is raised?
A. Caeruloplasmin
B. Complement proteins
C. Ferritin
D. Fibrinogen
E. All the above

Ans. E

6

MICROBIOLOGY AND IMMUNOLOGY

Choose the single best answer (SBA)

Q 1. Which of the following micro-organisms does not cause latent infection?
A. Cytomegalovirus (CMV)
B. Chlamydia trachomatis
C. Hepatitis A
D. Mycobacterium tuberculosis
E. Varicella zoster virus

Ans. C

Q 2. Which of the following micro-organisms is responsible for causing chronic osteomyelitis after implant surgery?
A. *Streptococcus pyogenes*
B. *Staphylococcus aureus*
C. *Haemophilus influenzae*
D. *Escherichia coli*
E. *Clostridium perfringens*

Ans. B

Q 3. Which of the following micro-organisms is responsible for causing pseudomembranous colitis?
A. *Streptococcus pyogenes*
B. *Clostridium difficile*
C. *Haemophilus influenzae*
D. *Escherichia coli*
E. *Clostridium perfringens*

Ans. B

Q 4. Which of the following is true regarding Neisseria?

A. *N. meningitidis* is a Gram-positive cocci
B. Infection with *N. gonorrhoeae* may cause suppurative urethritis in males
C. *N. gonorrhoeae* is a communal of the genital tract
D. *N. gonorrhoeae* thrives in conditions with low levels of carbon dioxide
E. Species cannot be cultured on chocolate agar

Ans. B

Q 5. Which of the following micro-organisms is responsible for causing gas gangrene?
A. *Streptococcus pyogenes*
B. *Clostridium difficile*
C. *Haemophilus influenzae*
D. *Escherichia coli*
E. *Clostridium perfringens*

Ans. E

Q 6. Which of the following is true regarding exotoxins?
A. Are derived from Gram-negative bacteria
B. Are more toxic than endotoxins
C. Are neutralised by their homologous antitoxin
D. Can be converted to a toxoid
E. All the above

Ans. E

Q 7. Which of the following statement is true regarding bacterial endotoxins?
A. Are components of the cell wall in Gram-negative bacteria
B. Are lipopolysaccharides
C. Induce fever
D. All the above
E. None of the above

Ans. D

Q 8. Which of the following is true regarding gonococcus?
A. Is a Gram-positive diplococcus bacillus
B. Is treated with erythromycin
C. Can penetrate the stratified squamous epithelium
D. It is insensitive to cold
E. In the male it may cause an acute suppurative urethritis and proctitis

Ans. E

Q 9. Which of the following is true regarding Clostridium tetani?
A. Causes gas gangrene
B. Has a sub-terminal spore
C. Is an obligatory anaerobe
D. Produces an endotoxin
E. It is non-motile

Ans. C

Q 10. The germination of tetanus spores in a wound is inhibited by which of the following?
A. Injection of anti-toxin
B. Injection of toxoid
C. Tissue trauma
D. Reduced blood supply
E. Decreased oxygen supply

Ans. B

Q 11. Which of the following is true regarding *Clostridium difficile* infection causing diarrhoea?
A. Successfully treated with intravenous vancomycin
B. More likely to develop with benzylpenicillin than third generation cephalosporins
C. Transmissible from person to person
D. Diagnosed by the isolation of Clostridium difficile from stool cultures

E. More likely to be community acquired than hospital acquired

Ans. C

Q 12. Which of the following antibiotics is usually effective against *Pseudomonas aeruginosa*?
A. Amoxicillin
B. Carbenicillin
C. Cephradine
D. Trimethoprim
E. Tetracycline

Ans. B

Q 13. Which of the following is not true concerning *Chlamydia trachomatis*?
A. Causes lymphogranuloma venereum
B. Causes non-specific urethritis
C. Is a precipitant of Reiter's syndrome
D. Treatment of choice is penicillin V
E. Is gram-negative bacteria

Ans. D

Q 14. Which of the following diseases are caused by Spirochaetes?
A. Bilharzia
B. Lymphogranuloma venereum
C. Weil's disease
D. Malaria
E. Chancroid

Ans. C

Q 15. *Treponema pallidum* immobilisation (TPI) test is positive in which of the following disease?
A. Chancroid
B. Infectious mononucleosis
C. Lyme disease (borreliosis)

D. Malaria
E. Yaws

Ans. E

Q 16. Which of the following is true regarding *Mycoplasma pneumoniae*?
A. Predominantly causes infection in the elderly
B. Can be grown on a cell-free medium
C. Infection is associated with a polymorphonuclear leucocytosis
D. White cell count is reduced
E. Infection is associated with the development of agglutinins to a haemolytic *Streptococcus*

Ans. B

Q 17. Which of the following diseases are caused by herpes simplex virus?
A. Cervical warts
B. Acute gingivostomatitis
C. Shingles
D. All the above
E. None of the above

Ans. B

Q 18. Which of the following group of viruses does the herpes group not include?
A. Cytomegalovirus
B. Epstein-Barr virus
C. Papilloma virus
D. Herpes simplex
E. Varicella-zoster virus

Ans. C

Q 19. Which of the following is true regarding the human papilloma virus?
A. It is a small RNA virus

B. It causes genital vesicles
C. It readily crosses the placenta
D. Effective vaccines now exist
E. It has a weak association with carcinoma cervix

Ans. D

Q 20. Which of the following is not true regarding Cytomegalovirus?
A. Causes haemolytic anaemia in the neonate
B. Is a cause of foetal cerebral calcification
C. Is an adenovirus
D. May be cultured readily in cell-free media
E. May be transmitted in saliva

Ans. C

Q 21. Which of the following is not true regarding sterilisation?
A. Ethylene oxide should only be used when heat sterilisation of an item is not possible
B. Flash autoclaving at 147ÅãC and 40 lb/square inch is no longer the preferred method of sterilisation by steam
C. Sterilisation by ethylene oxide has a broad-spectrum static action against bacteria, spores and viruses
D. Hot air sterilisation is the preferred method to treat surgical instruments with fine cutting edges
E. Unwrapped instruments may be sterilised in theatre using a portable steam steriliser

Ans. C

Q 22. Which of the following factor affects the performance of a disinfectant?
A. Concentration of disinfectant
B. Number of organisms present
C. pH
D. None of the above
E. All the above

Ans. E

Q 23. Which of the following does not reliably inactivate HIV?
A. Chlorhexidine
B. Glutaraldehyde
C. Hypochlorites
D. The autoclave
E. The hot-air oven

Ans. A

Q 24. Which of the following virus may exhibit oncogenic properties in humans?
A. Enteroviruses
B. Hepatitis B virus
C. Papovavirus
D. Rabies virus
E. Rubella virus

Ans. B

Q 25. Congenital abnormalities are not associated with which of the following maternal infections?
A. Hepatitis B
B. Group B streptococcus
C. Parvovirus
D. All the above
E. None of the above

Ans. D

Q 26. Which of the following is a Gram-negative bacteria?
A. *Lactobacillus acidophilus*
B. *Campylobacter jejuni*
C. *Clostridium difficile*
D. *Listeria monocytogenes*
E. *Staphylococcus aureus*

Ans. B

Q 27. Which of the following is true regarding immunoglobulins?
A. IgMs can cross the placenta to the foetus
B. Immunoglobulins are secreted from T-lymphocytes
C. IgG constitutes approximately 25% of all immunoglobulins in a healthy individual
D. The molecular structure of IgG is a Y shape
E. Secretion of immunoglobulins does not require response of a specific antigen

Ans. D

Q 28. Which of the following is true regarding immunoglobulin E (IgE)?
A. Present in normal serum in a concentration similar to that of IgG
B. Attached to mast cells in the skin
C. Involved in type II hypersensitivity mechanisms
D. Transmitted across the normal placenta
E. Found in low concentrations in the serum of patients with atopic eczema

Ans. B

Q 29. Which of the following is true regarding immunoglobulins?
A. Antiviral activity is provided mainly by IgA antibody
B. Immunoglobulins G are produced by T helper cells
C. All immunoglobulins are gamma-globulins
D. Immunoglobulin G (IgG) chains are coded for by adjacent genes on the same chromosome
E. Immunoglobulin A (IgA) is a cryoglobulin

Ans. A

Q 30. Concerning a hepatitis E infection, which of the following is true?
A. CT scan of the liver with contrast shows diagnostic appearances
B. It can be transmitted with hepatitis B

C. It is a recognised cause of chronic liver disease
D. The incidence of chronic liver disease is reduced by administration of alpha interferon
E. It does not result in a carrier state

Ans. E

7

GENETICS

Choose the single best answer (SBA)

Q 1. Which of the following statements regarding DNA is true?

A. Attached to the 2' position of the sugar ring is one of four bases
B. Guanine-cytosine bonds consist of three hydrogen bonds
C. The two strands of DNA separate in vitro by heating it to 75°C
D. All codons have an identical function
E. There is a greater variety of amino acids than there are different codons

Ans. B

Q 2. Which of the following statement is true regarding human chromosomes?
A. Banding with quinicrine fluorescent stain can be used to identify X chromosome
B. Banding can be used to determine polymorphism in populations
C. Telocentric chromosomes have a centrally placed centromere
D. Terminal fragments called 'satellites' are present in the metacentric chromosomes
E. Telocentric chromosomes are present in human

Ans. B

Q 3. The following are true regarding the Lyon's hypothesis
A. Lyon's hypothesis does not relate to germ cells
B. The inactivation of X chromosome usually occurs during 16 weeks of life
C. Barr body can be seen as a condensed mass during the prophase phase of mitosis
D. Barr body may be observed in up to 80% of cells on a buccal smear from a woman
E. Presence of an extra X chromosome is associated with

intelligence above average

Ans. A

Q 4. 46 XX karyotype is associated with which of the condition?
A. Testicular feminisation syndrome
B. Klinefelter's syndrome
C. Muscular dystrophy
D. Constitutional hirsutism
E. None of the above

Ans. D

Q 5. Which of the following is not associated with a karyotype of 46 XY?
A. Hydatidiform mole
B. Tay Sach's disease
C. Muscular dystrophy
D. All the above
E. None of the above

Ans. A

Q 6. Which of the following conditions is not associated with genetic anticipation?
A. Cystic fibrosis
B. Fragile X syndrome
C. Huntington's chorea
D. Myotonic dystrophy
E. None of the above

Ans. A

Q 7. Increased numbers of chromosomes occur in which of the following condition?
A. Fragile X syndrome
B. Down's syndrome
C. Phenylketonuria

D. Turners syndrome
E. Cri du chat syndrome

Ans. B

Q 8. Which of the following is not true regarding carriers of genetic disease?
A. Carrier state may be produced in an autosomal dominant
B. Certain carrier states can be detected using DNA studies
C. In case of cystic fibrosis if both the parents are carriers, the chances of having an affected child is 1 in 4
D. In X-linked genetic diseases, the female carriers may show certain disease manifestations
E. Marriage between the blood relatives is associated with an approximately double the risk of getting inherited disorders and birth defects

Ans. A

Q 9. Which of the following is true regarding Edward's syndrome?
A. Is characterised by the presence of three copies of chromosome 13
B. Has an autosomal recessive pattern of inheritance
C. There may be absence of femur
D. Increased space can be seen between the index and the middle finger
E. There may be only 11 pair of ribs

Ans. E

Q 10. Which of the following is true regarding Patau's Syndrome?
A. Is due to trisomy of chromosome 18
B. May be characterised by the presence of colobomas in the iris
C. There may be mild-to-moderate mental retardation
D. The infant's head may be abnormally large
E. Most individuals die within the first six months of life

Ans. B

Q 11. Which of the following is true regarding müllerian agenesis?
A. The ovaries are absent
B. The disease may be due to a genetic defect
C. Abnormalities of gastrointestinal tract are frequently present
D. Pubic/axillary hair are scanty or absent
E. Use of Franks dilators is an invasive form of therapy

Ans. B

Q 12. Which of the following is true regarding 5-α reductase deficiency
A. The disease is characterized by an abnormality of testosterone receptors
B. Dehydrotestosterone is not produced
C. The external genitalia develop normally
D. Has an X-linked inheritance
E. The karytotype is XXY
F. Breast development is like that of normal females

Ans. B

Q 13. Which of the following is true regarding Turner's syndrome?
A. The individual is phenotypically a female
B. Is associated with congenital absence of the uterus
C. Is associated with mental retardation
D. Has an autosomal recessive pattern of inheritance
E. Is associated with oestrogen insensitivity

Ans. A

Q 14. Which of the following disorders have an autosomal recessive pattern of inheritance?
A. Christmas disease
B. Neurofibromatosis
C. Colour blindness

D. Tay Sachs disease

E. Achondroplasia

Ans. D

Q 15. Which of the following disorders have an autosomal dominant pattern of inheritance?

A. Thalassaemia major

B. Galactosaemia

C. Polyposis coli

D. Vitamin D resistant rickets

E. Hemochromatosis

Ans. C

Q 16. Which of the following disorders have an X-linked mode of inheritance?

A. Adult polycystic kidney disease

B. Hurler's syndrome

C. Fragile X syndrome

D. Alzheimer's disease

E. Achondroplasia

Ans. C

Q 17. Which of the following statement regarding haemophilia A is correct?

A. Haemophilia A is commoner in females

B. If father is suffering from the disease and mother is the carrier of the abnormal gene, there is a 1 in 4 chance that the offspring will be affected

C. In mild cases bleeding must be controlled by the infusion of factor VIII

D. The increased bleeding tendency usually manifests after 1 year of age

E. Levels of factor VIII related antigen is normal in these cases

Ans. E

Q 18. Which of the following statement is true regarding Duchenne muscular dystrophy?

A. It shows an autosomal recessive pattern of inheritance
B. Is characterised by the weakness of distal muscles of leg
C. The affected father passes the defective gene to all his sons
D. Carrier mothers will always produce affected sons
E. Carrier mothers will have 50% probability of producing carrier daughters

Ans. E

Q 19. Which of the following statement is correct regarding McCune Albright syndrome?

A. Has an autosomal dominant pattern of inheritance
B. Can result in ovarian failure
C. There may be presence of neurofibromatas
D. Is associated with polyostotic fibrous dysplasia
E. Levels of gonadotropins are markedly reduced

Ans. D

Q 20. Which of the following statement regarding glucose-6-phosphate dehydrogenase deficiency is correct?

A. Shows an autosomal recessive pattern of inheritance
B. Can be triggered by ciprofloxacin
C. Can cause profound hypoglycaemia
D. Is common amongst Ashkenazi Jews
E. None of the above

Ans. B

Q 21. Which of the following statement regarding thalassemias is correct?

A. Shows X-linked recessive inheritance
B. There is marked reticulocytosis
C. There may be undergrowth of maxillary regions of face
D. There may be persistence of HbF
E. None of the above

Ans. D

Q 22. Which of the following statements regarding multifactorial inheritance is true?
A. Blood groups are inherited in this manner
B. Can be diagnosed by chromosome culture
C. It is due to the effects of a large number of gene and the environment
D. The recurrence risk in this type does not depend on the previous incidence of the same condition in the family.
E. None of the above

Ans. C

Q 23. Which of the following is not true regarding ambiguous external genitalia at birth?
A. Is associated with drug ingestion during pregnancy
B. Is commonly due to congenital adrenal hyperplasia
C. Occurs in true hermaphroditism
D. Occurs in complete testicular feminisation syndrome
E. There are normal male genitalia in 47,XXY Klinefelter's syndrome

Ans. D

Q 24. Which of the following is characteristically true concerning transexual patients?
A. Are of subnormal intelligence
B. Are socially well-adjusted
C. Have abnormal hormone profiles
D. Have abnormal karyotype
E. Have normal external genitalia

Ans. E

Q 25. Which of the following is true regarding hermaphroditism?
A. Chromosomal sex is usually female (46,XX)
B. End-organ resistance is a feature

C. External sex is usually female
D. Mosaics do not occur
E. Either the primordial follicles or the seminiferous tubules are present

Ans. A

Q 26. Which of the following statement concerning patients with pure gonadal dysgenesis is not correct?
A. Always have primary amenorrhoea
B. Are frequently XO or XO/mosaic
C. Have a uterus
D. Have LH and FSH concentrations within the normal range
E. Have poorly developed breasts

Ans. D

Q 27. Which of the following statement regarding genes is correct?
A. Introns are the portions of a gene which code for protein
B. Mitochondrial genes are inherited from the mother
C. Most of the human genome encodes polypeptide
D. The rate of DNA replication is directly under the control of enhancer sequences
E. Transcription factors are mainly made of DNA

Ans. B

Q 28. Which of the following is true concerning adenine?
A. Can be converted directly to a nucleotide by theaction of phosphoribosyl-transferase enzymes
B. Forms base pairs with thymine in RNA
C. Is a pyrimidine base
D. Is degraded by a pathway which involves the enzyme xanthine oxidase
E. Is synthesised attached to ribose phosphate

Ans. D

Q 29. Which of the following technique is not directly used for used for identifying DNA?
A. Denaturing gradient gel electrophoresis
B. Northern blotting
C. Polymerase chain reaction
D. Southern blotting
E. None of the above

Ans. D

Q 30. 46 XY karyotype is associated with which of the following condition?
A. MRKH syndrome
B. Testicular feminisation syndrome
C. Klinefelter's syndrome
D. All the above
E. None of the above

Ans. B

8

BIOPHYSICS

Choose the Single Best Answer (SBA)

Q 1. Children exposed in utero to X-ray irradiation are at an increased risk of which of the following?
A. Diabetes
B. Acute lymphoblastic leukaemia
C. Intra-uterine growth retardation (IUGR)
D. Mental retardation
E. None of the above

Ans. B

Q 2. Which of the following is true regarding diagnostic ultrasound?
A. Medical ultrasound uses the range of 1,000–5,000 kilohertz (kHz).
B. Is associated with a 1oC rise in body temperature after 15 minutes of scanning
C. It is ionising
D. It is pulsatile
E. High frequency ultrasound has greatest tissue penetration

Ans. D

Q 3. Which of the following is not true regarding ultrasound examination during pregnancy?
A. Can diagnose foetal ascites
B. Anomaly scanning is usually carried out in the second trimester of pregnancy
C. Cannot reliably establish foetal maturity at 34 weeks' gestation
D. Can diagnose a cleft lip
E. Is able to identify the fertilised ovum prior to implantation.

Ans. E

Q 4. In experimental conditions, which of the following biological effects can be produced on the tissues by the ultrasound waves?
A. Cavitation
B. Heat generation
C. Microstreaming
D. All the above
E. None of the above

Ans. D

Q 5. Which of the following statement regarding the properties of the ultrasound waves is not correct?
A. Impedance determines the proportion of sound energy reflected and transmitted at an interface
B. The size of a pulse generated in an A-scan is a measure of the intensity of the reflected ultrasonic echo
C. The sound travels poorly through air
D. The velocity is slower through a denser materials
E. The velocity is dependent on the temperature of the material through which it travels

Ans. D

Q 6. Which of the following statement is not correct regarding physics of ultrasound?
A. A thicker piezoelectric crystal has a longer wavelength
B. A thicker piezoelectric crystal has a lower resonance frequency
C. Acoustic impedance determines beam refraction
D. As the angle of incidence increases less sound is reflected
E. The acoustic impedance of a material is the product of its density and the velocity of sound within it
Ans. C

Q 7. Which of the following statement regarding the velocity of ultrasound is correct?

A. Is about 1540 m/s through the soft tissue
B. Is faster through air than water
C. Is faster through the soft tissue than the skull
D. Is proportional to the compressibility of the medium through which the sound travels
E. It is not dependent on the frequency

Ans. A

Q 8. Which of the following is true concerning a laser?
A. Is an acronym for Light Amplification of Stimulated Ejection of Radiation.
B. Produces multichromatic light
C. Requires a pair of mirrors at opposite ends of an optical cavity containing the lasing medium
D. The lasing medium can be gaseous or crystalline
E. The wavelength is determined by the stimulating current

Ans. C

Q 9. Which of the following classes of lasers is considered to be of low risk?
A. Class 3a
B. Class 3b
C. Class 4
D. None of the above
E. All the above

Ans. A

Q 10. Which of the following is true concerning MRI?
A. Blood vessels appear white on scanning
B. Has no recognised side effects on the foetus
C. It involves ionising radiation
D. The pregnant mother should be turned to her right side during scanning
E. Tissue with high hydrogen concentrations are difficult to distinguish

Ans. B

9

PHARMACOLOGY

Choose the Single Best Answer (SBA)

Q 1. Which of the following is true regarding clonidine?
  A. Is an alpha adrenergic receptor antagonist
  B. Does not cause dryness of mouth
  C. Reduces the minimal alveolar concentration of volatile anaesthetic agents
  D. Stimulates the release of catecholamines
  E. Sudden withdrawal is associated with hypotension

  Ans. C

Q 2. Which of the following substances are sympathomimetic amines?
  A. Ephedrine
  B. Amphetamine
  C. Isoprenaline
  D. None of the above
  E. All of the above

  Ans. E

Q 3. Which of the following is not true regarding the drugs acting on the uterus?
  A. Ergometrine is an oxytocic
  B. Prostaglandin F2α may lead to an elevation of blood pressure
  C. Oxytocin is a nonapeptide hormone
  D. Mifepristone is an antiprogestogenic steroid
  E. Ergometrine has a greater effect on the uterus at term than in early pregnancy

  Ans. B

Q 4. Calcium antagonists are not used for treating which of the following diseases?

A. Angina
B. Hypertension
C. Pulmonary hypertension
D. Raynaud's phenomenon
E. Thyrotoxicosis

Ans. E

Q 5. Which of the following statements is not correct regarding the antibiotics?
A. Metronidazole given by the rectal route is as effective as when given by the intravenous route
B. Streptomycin is nephrotoxic
C. Aminoglycosides are effective against anaerobes
D. Ampicillin may potentiate the anticoagulant effect of warfarin
E. Rifampicin use is not associated with an increased risk of neonatal bleeding in the third trimester

Ans. E

Q 6. Which of the following micro-organisms are sensitive to benzylpenicillin?

A. *Bordetella pertussis*
B. *Cryptococcus neoformans*
C. *Mycoplasma pneumoniae*
D. *All the above*
E. *None of the above*

Ans. E

Q 7. Resistance to penicillin is present in over 20% of isolates of which of the following bacterial species?
A. *Escherichia coli*
B. *Haemophilus influenzae*

C. *Neisseria meningitides*
D. Beta-haemolytic *Streptococci*
E. *Pseudomonas aeruginosa*

Ans. A

Q 8. Which of the following is true regarding penicillins?

A. Are bacteriostatic
B. Exert their actions by combining with a transpeptidase
C. Have a spectrum of action, which is independent of the beta lactam side chain
D. Have significant toxic effects on humans
E. Are not inactivated by the plasmid coded enzymes

Ans. B

Q 9. Which of the following is not true regarding co-trimoxazole?

A. Contains two different drugs
B. Displaces methotrexate from protein binding sites
C. Inhibits folic acid synthesis
D. Is bacteriostatic
E. Potentiates the action of warfarin

Ans. D

Q 10. Which of the following is true concerning carbimazole?

A. Is not a prodrug
B. Is contraindicated in breast feeding and pregnant mothers
C. Is teratogenic
D. May cause lymphadenopathy
E. May cause irreversible agranulocytosis

Ans. D

Q 11. Which of the following is true regarding suxamethonium?

A. Ecothiophate shortens its duration of action
B. Is a non-depolarising muscle relaxant
C. May be reversed using neostigmine
D. May trigger anaphylaxis
E. Has a shorter duration of action in pregnancy

Ans. D

Q 12. Which of the following statements is not true regarding low molecular weight heparin?

A. Exerts its anticoagulant effect by binding with antithrombin
B. Has fewer chains containing the unique pentasaccharide sequence (the binding site) than unfractionated heparin
C. Is excreted in the urine
D. Binds less to platelets, endothelium and von Willibrand factor
E. Inactivates thrombin more readily than unfractionated heparin

Ans. E

Q 13. Which of the following is true regarding heparin?
A. Enhances antithrombin III activity
B. Has no effect on platelet aggregation
C. Induces thrombocytopenia in 20% of patients
D. Is a strongly acidic protein
E. Readily crosses the placenta

Ans. A

Q 14. Which of the following does not have an anti-emetic action?

A. Chloropropamide
B. Hyoscine hydrobromide

C. Morphine sulphate
D. Perphenazine
E. Promethazine hydrochloride

Ans. C

Q 15. Which of the following is a physiological effect of metoclopramide?

A. Acts on central dopaminergic receptors
B. Increases gastric acid secretion
C. Increases gastric fluid pH
D. Decreases gastroesophageal sphincter tone
E. Inhibits upper gastrointestinal motility

Ans. A

Q 16. Which of the following statements is true regarding domperidone?

A. Is not a recognised cause of galactorrhoea
B. Is less likely to produce acute dystonia than metoclopramide
C. Is typically associated with parkinsonian-like adverse effects
D. Protects against drug-induced vomiting if given five minutes after apomorphine
E. Inhibits gastric peristalsis

Ans. B

Q 17. Ondansetron probably mediate its antiemetic effects by interacting with which of the following receptor systems?

A. Dopaminergic
B. GABA
C. Muscarinic/cholinergic
D. Nicotinic/cholinergic
E. Serotinergic

Ans. E

Q 18. Which of the following is not true concerning diazepam?

    A. Effects may be antagonised by flumazenil
    B. Has a hypnotic effect
    C. Has an anticonvulsant effect
    D. Has an antidepressant effect
    E. Is a respiratory depressant

Ans. D

Q 19. Which of the following antihypertensives are ACE inhibitors?

    A. Lisinopril
    B. Losartan
    C. Propranolol
    D. All the above
    E. None of the above

Ans. A

Q 20. Which of the following side-effects can occur as a result of glucocorticoid therapy?

    A. Hypertrichosis
    B. Hypokalaemia
    C. Lymphopenia
    D. All the above
    E. None of the above

Ans. D

Q 21. Which of the following statement is correct regarding the antiviral drugs?
    A. Zidovudine eliminates the HIV virus
    B. Inosine pranobex enhances the B-cell response to many viruses, including herpes and HIV

C. High levels of beta-interferon are found in the amniotic fluid and in the placenta
D. Acyclovir prevents DNA synthesis
E. Amantadine does not have an adverse effect on breastfeeding.

Ans. D

Q 22. Which of the following agents interfere with viral multiplication?
A. Amantadine
B. Ribavirin
C. Zidovudine
D. None of the above
E. All the above

Ans. E

Q 23. Which of the following are antiplatelet agents?

A. Heparin
B. Nitric oxide
C. Warfarin
D. None of the above
E. All of the above

Ans. B

Q 24. Which of the following is true concerning labetalol?

A. Causes bronchodilation
B. Decreases bile secretion
C. Has a half life of 2 hours
D. Has only alpha blocking action
E. Is 70% protein bound

Ans. B

Q 25. Which of the following are known complications of phenytoin therapy?
  A. Alopecia
  B. Dental caries
  C. Balding
  D. Microcytic anemia
  E. None of the above

  Ans. A

Q 26. Which of the following is true regarding propranolol?

  A. Crosses the blood brain barrier poorly
  B. Has a long elimination half-life
  C. Has a small volume of distribution
  D. Exacerbates bronchospasm
  E. Is a cardio-selective beta adrenoceptor antagonist

  Ans. D

Q 27. Which of the following are potassium-sparing diuretics?

  A. Bendroflumethiazide
  B. Captopril
  C. Furosemide
  D. Triamterene
  E. None of the above

  Ans. D

Q 28. Which of the following drug in pharmacological doses have been shown to cause a rise in blood glucose?
  A. Thiazide diuretics
  B. Ethanol
  C. Aspirin
  D. Gliclazide
  E. Atenolol

Ans. A

Q 29. Which of the following are true regarding cabergoline?

    A. Has a half-life of 8 hours
    B. Is a dopamine antagonist
    C. Is an effective antiemetic
    D. Is not used during pregnancy
    E. May cause parkinsonian side effects

    Ans. D

Q 30. Which of the following is true concerning lidocaine?
    A. Inhibits the conduction of neuronal impulses
    B. Inhibits the generation of neuronal impulse
    C. Is associated with haemolytic anaemia
    D. Is effective for the treatment of both supraventricular and ventricular tachycardia
    E. Is only effective via oral route

    Ans. A

10

OBSTETRICS AND GYNAECOLOGY

Choose the single best answer (SBA)

Q 1. Which of the following statement is not correct regarding miscarriage?
A. If recurrent, it can be associated with parental chromosomal translocation.
B. If recurrent, it can be associated with sickle cell trait.
C. The clinical diagnosis of incomplete miscarriage is assisted by digital examination of the cervical canal.
D. Cervical incompetence causes recurrent second trimester miscarriage.
E. Missed miscarriage should be suspected if the uterine size is smaller than that expected for gestational age.

Ans. B

Q 2. Which of the following statement is correct regarding the early pregnancy loss?
A. Is usually due to hormone deficiency.
B. Is due to an abnormal karyotype in approximately 5% of cases.
C. Intrauterine pregnancy cannot co-exist with tubal pregnancy.
D. An intrauterine pregnancy should be visible on transvaginal scan if the HCG is > 1,000 i.u./l.
E. Always needs evacuation.

Ans. D

Q 3. Which of the following is true regarding threatened miscarriage at eight weeks of gestation?
A. The prognosis can be determined in most cases by ultrasound.
B. Can be effectively treated with depot progestogens

C. Always needs evacuation if non-viable
D. Anti-D immunoglobulin should be administered if the mother is Rhesus negative.
E. May co-exist with ectopic pregnancy

Ans. E

Q 4. Which of the following is not true concerning thalassaemia in pregnancy?
A. Thalassaemia minor may be suspected on a blood film.
B. Thalassaemia is particularly concentrated in a broad band encompassing the Mediterranean and Middle East.
C. The carrier rate in the UK is approximately 1 in 10,000.
D. A woman with α-thalassaemia minor can be reassured that the baby will be healthy.
E. Presence of thalassaemia trait has no association with the occurrence of preeclampsia.

Ans. D

Q 5. Which of the following is not true regarding intrauterine growth restriction?
A. It is associated with premature labour
B. It may be associated with a low socio-economic status
C. These babies are at an increased risk of developing respiratory distress syndrome
D. It may be associated with raised serum AFP at 16 weeks followed by normal scan at18 weeks
E. There may be neonatal hypoglycaemia in the babies born with IUGR

Ans. A

Q 6. Which of the following is not correct concerning maternal cardiac disease in pregnancy?
A. A classification system exists to determine the mortality risk.
B. Involvement of the aorta in Marfan's syndrome increases the

mortality.

C. The foetus has an increased risk of congenital heart disease.

D. Mitral stenosis is an infrequent complication following rheumatic heart disease.

E. Women with primary pulmonary hypertension should be advised against pregnancy.

Ans. D

Q 7. Which of the following is true regarding thyrotoxicosis in pregnancy?
A. It is usually due to a solitary adenoma
B. The major maternal risk is congestive cardiac failure
C. Beta-blocking drugs are contra-indicated
D. May be treated with radioactive iodine as the drug does not cross the placenta
E. Usually occurs as new disease as a result of HCG stimulation of the thyroid

Ans. B

Q 8. Which of the following is not true regarding thyroid disease in pregnancy?
A. Hyperthyroidism may be associated with IUGR
B. Thiouracil may cause severe liver disease
C. Congenital hypothyroidism is not routinely screened for in the UK
D. Thyrotoxicosis is associated with increased hepatic metabolism of "the Pill"
E. Raised T3 and T4 levels are found in hyperemesis and molar pregnancy

Ans. C

Q 9. Which of the following is true regarding the monozygotic twins?
A. Are more common than dizygotic twins
B. Are commonly familial

C. May be reliably distinguished from dizygotic twins by the naked-eye examination of the fetal membranes and placentae
D. Have a higher incidence of placenta praevia than singleton pregnancies
E. Are associated with oligohydramnios.

Ans. D

Q 10. Which of the following complication is associated with multiple births?
A. Increased incidence of congenital abnormalities
B. Increased incidence of growth retardation
C. Increased incidence of postpartum haemorrhage
D. Increased incidence of preterm labour
E. All the above

Ans. E

Q 11. Which of the following statement is not correct regarding preeclampsia?
A. The perinatal mortality is raised
B. Epigastric pain may indicate impending eclampsia
C. There are lowered serum urate levels
D. There may be no foetus
E. The liquor volume may be diminished.

Ans. C

Q 12. Which of the following is required for the diagnosis of pre-eclampsia?
A. High urate levels
B. Low plasma magnesium levels
C. More than 24 weeks gestation
D. Oedema
E. Proteinuria

Ans. E

Q 13. Which of the following features is compatible with hypertension?
A. A fourth heart sound
B. A soft aortic second heart sound
C. Retinal haemorrhages and soft exudates, indicating a grade 2 hypertensive retinopathy
D. A tapping apex beat
E. A third heart sound

Ans. A

Q 14. Which of the following is not true regarding placental abruption?
A. May have no associated vaginal bleeding
B. Is an indication for delivery
C. Has a higher incidence with maternal cocaine abuse
D. May be identified using ultrasound to demonstrate retroplacental clot
E. The diagnosis of concealed abruption can be easily confused with that of acute appendicitis.

Ans. B

Q 15. Which of the following is true regarding ABO incompatibility between mother and the foetus?
A. May affect the first pregnancy.
B. Worsens with successive pregnancies
C. Usually causes significant anaemia of the foetus at birth.
D. Often requires exchange transfusion.
E. Is caused by the Rh(D) antigen.

Ans. A

Q 16. Which of the following is not true regarding ABO blood group incompatibility between mother and foetus?
A. It is associated with a strongly positive direct Coombs' test
B. Its severity does not vary between the first and subsequent pregnancies
C. It is usually detected in the antenatal period

D. Manifests itself on the first or second day of life

E. Affects only the first pregnancy

Ans. E

Q 17. Which of the following does not occur in uncomplicated haemolytic jaundice?

A. High levels of urobilinogen

B. High levels of unconjugated serum bilirubin

C. High serum alkaline phosphatase

D. Reticulocytosis

E. Urobilinuria

Ans. C

Q 18. Which of the following is correct regarding the neonatal jaundice?

A. Early onset usually indicates a haemolytic process

B. May be due to sickle cell disease

C. Is more common after forceps delivery compared with the ventouse

D. Mild cases may benefit from ultraviolet light

E. May be due to glucose 6 phosphatase deficiency

Ans. A

Q 19. Which of the following statement is true regarding monilial infection?

A. Is due to a flagellate organism.

B. Responds to metronidazole.

C. Is a common presenting feature in juvenile diabetes.

D. The organisms are commonly present in asymptomatic women.

E. Fluconazole is of proven safety in pregnancy.

Ans. D

Q 20. Which of the following is true regarding colposuspension?

A. Is normally done as a vaginal procedure

B. Is effective in relieving urge incontinence.

C. Is effective in relieving dyspareunia
D. Is associated with an increased incidence of posterior vaginal wall prolapse
E. Cannot be done via the laparoscope

Ans. D

Q 21. Which of the following is not true regarding genital warts?
A. They are always sexually transmitted
B. Additional cervical screening is not justified, provided that the woman has had a screening test within the previous 3–5 years
C. Podophyllin paint cannot be used with safety during pregnancy
D. Condom usage with regular sex partners has not been shown to affect the treatment outcome
E. All treatments have significant failure and relapse rates

Ans. A

Q 22. Which of the following procedures does not help correct retroversion of the uterus?
A. Hodge pessary
B. A laparoscopic procedure
C. A sling operation
D. Pelvic floor repair
E. Gilliam's operation

Ans. D

Q 23. Which of the following is true regarding myomectomy?
A. Is an underused alternative to hysterectomy
B. Is useful in the management of infertility
C. Is useful in managing menorrhagia
D. Makes Caesarean section obligatory in subsequent pregnancy
E. None of the above

Ans. E

Q 24. Which of the following is true regarding colposuspension for treatment of uterine retroversion?

A. Effectively treats dyspareunia
B. Effectively treats frequency of micuturition
C. Is an appropriate treatment for enterocoele
D. Is associated with a need to treat rectocoele
E. Is usually performed vaginally

Ans. D

Q 25. Which of the following statement is not correct regarding the mobile retroversion of the uterus?
A. It is suspected when the cervix points anteriorly on speculum examination
B. Is usually asymptomatic
C. Occurs at 20 weeks gestation
D. May occur in 20% of women
E. Occurs in the puerperium

Ans. C

Q 26. Which of the following changes does not commonly occur in uterine leiomyomata?
A. Atrophy
B. Calcification
C. Hyaline degeneration
D. Squamous metaplasia
E. Sarcomatous change

Ans. D

Q 27. Which of the following is not correct regarding the masses of ovarian origin?
A. Include benign teratomas
B. Those of germ cell origin may secrete hormones
C. Are always malignant in the presence of ascites
D. May be confused with developmental abnormalities of the renal tract
E. Careful surgical staging is essential to determine the appropriate subsequent management

Ans. C

Q 28. Which of the following is true regarding central parenteral nutrition?
A. Does not cause derangement of liver function tests
B. Is a hypo-osmolar solution
C. Is not associated with any metabolic disturbance
D. Typically contains about 250 g glucose
E. Typically contains 14–16 g nitrogen as D-amino acids

Ans. D

Q 29. Which of the following is true regarding hirsutism?
A. Is synonymous with virilisation
B. Is pathological in most cases
C. Is a side effect of cyproterone
D. Androgens in women are produced solely in the adrenal
E. May be due to an ovarian tumour

Ans. E

Q 30. Dyspareunia may result from which of the following?
A. Adenomyosis
B. The climacteric
C. Superficial vulvovaginitis
D. All the above
E. None of the above

Ans. D

MODEL TEST PAPER 1

Time alloted: 2.5 hours

Q 1. Which of the following statements concerning the reporting of adverse drug reactions (ADR) in the United Kingdom is not correct?

A. A black triangle sign alongside a drug within the British National Formulary (BNF) requires that all ADRs should be reported with this drug
B. ADR reporting is compulsory
C. Reporting is required for ADRs associated with vaccinations
D. There is a requirement to report ADRs with over the counter (OTC) drugs as well
E. When submitting a yellow card concerning an ADR, all other drugs taken within the last 3 months should also be reported

Ans. B

Q 2. Which of the following is not correct regarding the detection of β-hCG levels during early pregnancy?

A. Levels which rise less than 50% in 48 hours at 6 weeks may indicate ectopic pregnancy
B. Levels > 8,000 i.u./l with no scan evidence of an intrauterine pregnancy strongly suggest ectopic pregnancy
C. Levels < 1,000 i.u./l at 8 weeks suggest ectopic pregnancy or pregnancy failure
D. Levels are above normal in hydatidiform mole
E. None of the above

Ans. D

Q 3. "A neonate is admitted to the hospital at 14 days of life with

the complaints of failure to thrive, tachypnoea and difficulty in feeding. He is diagnosed as having a circulatory defect."
Administration of prostaglandin antagonists soon after birth can be used for therapeutic closure of which patent structure of foetal origin?
A. Ductus venosus
B. Foramen ovale
C. Ductus arteriosus
D. Fossa ovalis
E. Ligamentum venosum

Ans. C

Q 4. Erythrocyte sedimentation rate (ESR) is increased in the following circumstances?
A. Following the infusion of high-molecular-weight dextran
B. In men compared with women
C. In polycythaemia rubra vera
D. Increase in the plasma fibrinogen concentrations
E. In young age

Ans. D

Q 5. A 65-years-old woman presented to the GP with the complaints of abdominal distension, reduced appetite and shortness of breath. The GP, suspicious of malignancy, referred her to the oncology department of the local hospital and ordered CA-125 levels.
CA-125 levels were found to be 820 U/mL. What is the likely diagnosis in this case?
A. Colorectal cancer
B. Hepatocellular cancer
C. Gastric cancer
D. Primary peritoneal cancer
E. Pancreatic cancer

Ans. D

Q 6. Which of the following is true regarding haemoglobin

values of less 10g/dL during pregnancy?
  A. Is a recognised side-effect of anti-convulsant therapy
  B. Is associated with urinary tract infection
  C. Is a complication of multiple pregnancy
  D. Increases the risk of post-partum haemorrhage
  E. All the above

Ans. E

Q 7. Which of the following is true concerning sickle cell disorders in pregnancy?
  A. Sickle cell disorders are most common in women of Asian origin.
  B. A sickle cell crisis can be precipitated in conditions of heightened oxygen tension.
  C. Sickle cell disorders are associated with an increased incidence of hypertension during pregnancy.
  D. Sickle cell disease results from a variant on the alpha globin chain.
  E. Partner screening is recommended during the second trimester

Ans. C

Q 8. Which of the following statement is not true regarding the perinatal mortality rate?
  A. It is usually expressed at the rate per thousand total births over one year
  B. It is attributable to congenital malformations in 50% of cases
  C. In England and Wales, it is higher in those whose mother was born in Pakistan than in those whose mother was born in the West Indies
  D. The rate is marginally higher in boys
  E. It is lowest in mothers aged between 20 and 29 years

Ans. B

Q 9. Which of the following is an essential amino acid?
A. Arginine

B. Methionine
C. Glycine
D. Tryptophan
E. Valine

Ans. B

Q 10. Which of the following statement is correct regarding obstetric cholestasis (OC)?
    A. OC usually presents with jaundice.
    B. Ursodeoxycholic acid is recommended to reduce foetal risk.
    C. Dexamethasone is recommended to reduce fetal and maternal risk.
    D. The symptoms of OC can recur if an affected woman takes the pill
    E. The risk of recurrence in a subsequent pregnancy is a rare event

    Ans. D

Q 11. A 50-year-old man is receiving anti-coagulant therapy (warfarin, a vitamin K antagonist) after heart valve replacement. He is admitted to hospital with haematuria (blood in the urine) and his INR (international normalised ratio, a measure of the prothrombin clotting time in relation to the normal time) is found to be 4.2. What is the most likely abnormality to be revealed by the laboratory investigations in this case?
A. Deficiency of vitamin K
B. Deficiency of factor VIII
C. Increased fibrinogen level
D. Platelet count 20 x 10^9 per litre
E. Deficiency of prothrombin

Ans. E

Q 12. Which of the following is true regarding folic acid?
A. Is a fat-soluble vitamin
B. Requires gastric intrinsic factor for its absorption

C. Is necessary for nucleic acid synthesis
D. Is heat-stable
E. Is involved in the tricarboxylic acid (Kreb's) cycle

Ans. C

Q 13. What is the most appropriate treatment option in an 8-week pregnant woman with vaginal candida infection unresponsive to clotrimazole cream?
    A. Metronidazole 400 mg orally
    B. Fluconazole 400 mg
    C. Hydrocortisone cream 0.5%
    D. Trimovate cream
    E. Clotrimazole pessary

    Ans. E

Q 14. What is the anticoagulant of choice in a pregnant woman with previous history of multiple pulmonary embolisms at 8 weeks of gestation?
    A. Aspirin 500 mg
    B. Heparin infusion
    C. Low-molecular weight heparin
    D. Warfarin
    E. Aspirin 300 mg

    Ans. C

Q 15. A typical lymphocytosis is not a feature of which of the following diseases?
A. Cytomegalovirus (CMV) infection
B. Epstein-Barr virus (EBV) infection
C. Influenza B infection
D. Rubella infection
E. Toxoplasmosis

Ans. C

Q 16. Which of the following is true regarding hypertension in

pregnancy?
- A. It is of little significance unless accompanied by proteinuria
- B. It causes foetal growth restriction in more than half of affected women
- C. It is not associated with an increased incidence of bleeding from placental praevia
- D. It should be assessed by admission to hospital
- E. It is a contraindication to the use of intramuscular ergometrine.

Ans. E

Q 17. Which of the following statement is correct regarding Conn's syndrome?
- A. Is caused by squamous cell carcinoma of adrenal glands
- B. Is characterized by profound hypotension
- C. Shows no response to spironolactone
- D. Is associated with excessive production of aldosterone
- E. Can cause hyperkalemia

Ans. D

Q 18. Which of the following vulval skin disorders is associated with the highest risk of malignancy?
- A. Lichen planus
- B. Lichen sclerosus
- C. Psoriasis
- D. Squamous cell metaplasia
- E. Contact irritant dermatitis

Ans. B

Q 19. Which of the following is true regarding hysterosalpingography?
- A. It should be performed in the luteal phase of the menstrual cycle
- B. It requires the use of ultrasound
- C. It may be used for investigating both primary and secondary subfertility
- D. A pregnancy test may be required before the procedure

E. It is contraindicated in the individuals with the history of Chlamydia

Ans. C

Q 20. Pulmonary surfactant increases which of the following?
A. The surface tension of the fluid lining alveolar walls
B. Lung compliance
C. In effectiveness as the lungs are inflated
D. In amount when pulmonary blood flow is interrupted
E. Breathing difficulties in the foetuses during the last month of pregnancy

Ans. B

Q 21. Circulating red blood cells
A. Are about 1 percent nucleated
B. May show an intracellular network pattern if appropriately stained
C. Are distributed evenly across the blood stream in large blood vessels
D. Travel at slower velocity in venules than in capillaries
E. Can easily pass through the capillaries without undergoing any deformation

Ans. B

Q 22. The standard chest X-ray is equivalent to what duration of natural background radiation?
    A. 7–10 days
    B. 10 days
    C. 2 months
    D. 10 months
    E. 2 years

    Ans. A

Q 23. Which of the following is true regarding bicornuate uterus?
    A. Is the commonest cause of unstable lie

B. Should be treated surgically if pregnancy has resulted in premature delivery
C. Is associated with premature labour
D. Is a proven cause of recurrent miscarriage
E. is associated with placental abruption

Ans. C

Q 24. A 16-year-old girl has primary dysmenorrhoea. Which is the most suitable treatment in this case?
A. D&C
B. Paracervical block
C. Non-steroidal anti-inflammatory drugs
D. GnRH analogue
E. Laser ablation of the endometrium

Ans. C

Q 25. A team wishes to audit their departmental results on the use of anticoagulation in patients with obstetric thromboembolic disease. What is the most appropriate next step to be taken up by the team who is undertaking audit in this case?
A. Data analysis
B. Data collection
C. Identify standards
D. Implement change
E. Needs assessment

Ans. C

Q 26. Which of the following is/are true concerning the oxygen dissociation curve (ODC)?
A. At 75% saturation the PO_2 is 40 mmHg (5.3 kPa)
B. Is hyperbolic in shape
C. Is shifted to the left by increase in 2,3-DPG
D. Is shifted to the right in methaemoglobinaemia
E. The Bohr effect shifts the curve to the left

Ans. A

Q 27. Which of the following statement regarding opioid drugs is correct?
A. Cause pupillary dilation
B. Lead to a decrease in the release of vasopressin
C. Cannot cross the placenta
D. Codeine is more potent analgesic than dihydrocodeine
E. Morphine can cause hypotension associated with a reflex tachycardia

Ans. D

Q 28. Which of the following is true regarding GnRH?
A. It is distinct from LH-RH
B. It is produced in the posterior pituitary
C. It is a decapeptide
D. It exerts its main effect directly on the ovary
E. It is used for inducing ovulation in IVF programmes

Ans. C

Q 29. A 25-year-old female presents with postnatal depression and refuses treatment. What is the most suitable form of consent, which must be obtained in this case?
A. Consent from carer
B. Consent from court of law
C. Consent from next of kin if possible
D. Verbal consent required
E. No consent required

Ans. C

Q 30. Which of the following is true concerning intermenstrual bleeding (IMB)?
A. IMB occurs in about 10% of normal menstrual cycles.
B. Laparoscopy should be included as part of the investigation.
C. A luteal phase progesterone is essential.
D. IMB may be associated with ovulation.
E. IMB is a feature of cervical intra-epithelial neoplasia.

Ans. D

Q 31. Which of the following is not true regarding submucous uterine fibroids?
A. Can become infected
B. Frequently cause infertility
C. May become polypoidal
D. May protrude through the cervix
E. Often present with menorrhagia

Ans. B

Q 32. Which of the following substances can be reabsorbed from the renal tubule?
A. Creatinine
B. Inulin
C. Mannitol
D. Sucrose
E. Urea

Ans. E

Q 33. Which of the following is true regarding uterine fibroids?
A. Undergo malignant degeneration in 5% of cases
B. If present in pregnancy, myomectomy should be performed at 14 weeks to prevent "red degeneration" later in pregnancy
C. Can be effectively treated with an LH-RH analogue
D. Commonly co-exist with endometriosis
E. Are a common cause of acute retention of urine

Ans. D

Q 34. Which of the following is not correct concerning the electrocardiogram (ECG) of an adult human?
A. A PR interval of 0.3 seconds indicates impaired conduction
B. During the isoelectric phase between the S and T waves, the intracellular potential in ventricular muscle cells is positive with respect to the interstitial fluid
C. Normal QT interval is 0.5s

D. The Q wave coincides with repolarisation of the atria

E. The R wave coincides with depolarisation of the apex of the heart

Ans. E

Q 35. Which of the following symptoms is characteristically associated with uterine fibromyomata?

    A. Abdominal pain

    B. Dysmenorrhoea

    C. Dyspareunia

    D. Menorrhagia

    E. Vaginal discharge

    Ans. D

Q 36. Which of the following characteristics about rectus sheath is correct?

A. Below the arcuate line, the posterior layer of the rectus sheath is formed by the transversalis fascia.

B. Each rectus abdominis muscle is attached by a single tendon to the pubic bone.

C. Below the arcuate line, the posterior wall of the sheath is formed by internal oblique.

D. All the above

E. None of the above

Ans. A

Q 37. What is the main site of vitamin B12 absorption?

A. Stomach

B. Upper small intestine

C. Lower small intestine

D. Colon

E. Rectum

Ans. C

Q 38. Gastric juice deficiency is likely to result in which of the following abnormality?

A. Pale stools
B. Local infections
C. Steatorrhoea
D. Milk intolerance
E. Anaemia

Ans. E

Q 39. Gonococcus can be found in which of the following tissues?
  A. Anus
  B. Endocervix
  C. Endometrium
  D. Epididymis
  E. All the above

  Ans. E

Q 40. Which of the following viruses cannot be sexually transmitted?
  A. Echovirus
  B. Hepatitis B
  C. Herpes simplex virus
  D. Papovavirus
  E. None of the above

  Ans. A

Q 41. Which of the following is not a side effect of alpha methyldopa?
  A. Depression
  B. Nasal congestion
  C. Oedema
  D. Pyrexia
  E. Visual disturbances

  Ans. E

Q 42. At a recent directorate meeting, an obstetrician has been nominated to undertake the next clinical audit. What is the most appropriate next step for the team undertaking audit in this

case?
  A. Data analysis
  B. Data collection
  C. Needs assessment
  D. Identify standards
  E. Implement change

Ans. C

Q 43. Which of the following organisms is not a common cause of urinary tract infection?
  A. *Candida*
  B. *Chlamydia*
  C. *Enterobacter*
  D. *Klebsiella*
  E. *Proteus*

Ans. B

Q 44. Which of the following is true regarding the development of the female genital tract and genitalia?
A. Sexual differentiation of the external genitalia is complete by 10 weeks
B. The clitoris is derived from the genital tubercle
C. The external genitalia only change under the influence of oestrogens produced by the placenta
D. The urogenital sinus forms the lower 1/3 of the vagina
E. The uterus and upper 2/3 of the vagina are derived from the paramesonephric ducts

Ans. B

Q 45. In the femoral triangle, which of the following is/are true of the femoral artery?
A. Crossed by the superficial circumflex iliac vein
B. Lateral to the femoral nerve
C. Medial to the long saphenous vein
D. Posterior to the femoral branch of the genitofemoral nerve
E. Posterior to the femoral vein at the apex of the triangle

Ans. D

Q 46. Which of the following structures pass under the inguinal ligament?
A. The long saphenous vein
B. The superficial femoral artery
C. The superficial epigastric vein
D. The genital branch of the genitofemoral nerve
E. The femoral branch of the genitofemoral nerve

Ans. E

Q 47. Which of the following is true concerning the femoral ring?
A. It is bounded laterally by the femoral artery.
B. It is bounded medially by the lacunar ligament.
C. It is lined by peritoneum.
D. It is not traversed by lymph vessels.
E. Passes deep to the inguinal ligament.

Ans. B

Q 48. Which of the following regarding thyroid function is true during normal pregnancy?
A. Foetal thyroid function is largely dependent upon the function of the maternal thyroid
B. Plasma thyroid-binding globulin concentration increases
C. Plasma total thyroxine concentration falls
D. Plasma TSH concentration increases
E. Tri-iodothyronine is not able to cross the placenta to the foetus

Ans. B

Q 49. Which of the following antibiotics is suitable for treating *Escherichia coli*?

A. Cefuroxime
B. Ciprofloxacin

C. Co-amoxiclav
D. All the above
E. None of the above

Ans. D

Q 50. Which of the following drugs are not accepted to be safe for treating pregnancy hypertension?
A. Nifedipine
B. Hydralazine
C. Magnesium sulphate
D. Methyl dopa
E. Diuretics

Ans. E

Q 51. Second trimester bleeding may be due to which of the following cause?
A. Missed abortion
B. Premature labour
C. Erythroblastosis fetalis
D. Threatened abortion
E. Monilial infection

Ans. D

Q 52. Which of the following is correct regarding vitamin B12?
A. Is a fat-soluble vitamin
B. Absorption takes place throughout the small intestine
C. Is essential for the metabolism of folic acid in the human
D. Deficiency leads to microcytic anaemia
E. Deficiency is common in non-vegetarians

Ans. C

Q 53. Which of the following is true regarding electrosurgery?
A. Bipolar diathermy can be used for cutting tissues
B. Monopolar diathermy necessitates the use of a return electrode

C. Diathermy uses low-frequency alternating current
D. Desiccation of the tissues is achieved only via bipolar diathermy and not by unipolar diathermy
E. Direct coupling is achieved by adhering to strict safety protocols

Ans. B

Q 54. Which of the following is true regarding asymptomatic bacteriuria (ASB)?
A. Should be investigated postpartum by IVP
B. Ascending infection occurs in about 30% of pregnant women with ASB
C. A significant count is more than 106 organisms per mL of urine
D. Is usually due to chlamydia
E. Screening should be by microscopy and culture of a "clean catch" urine specimen, not dipsticks

Ans. B

Q 55. In cases of non-gonococcal urethritis (NGU), which of the following statement is correct?
A. Association with septic arthritis is common
B. *Chlamydia trachomatis* is the commonest organism
C. Chronic conjunctivitis is not a recognised sequel
D. Cystitis is typical
E. It is usually treated with Septrin

Ans. B

Q 56. Whilst examining the abdomen of a 21-year-old female with abdominal pain you notice a welldefined "six-pack". Which muscle is this?
A. Rectus abdominis
B. Transversus abdominis
C. Cremaster
D. External oblique
E. Internal oblique

Ans. A

Q 57. Which of the following is true concerning the Müllerian ducts?
A. Are derived from coelomic epithelium
B. Form the vas deferens
C. Form urogenital sinus in their lowest part
D. Fuse from above downwards
E. Grow medial to the Wolffian ducts

Ans. A

Q 58. Which of the following muscles develops from the second pharyngeal arch?
A. Anterior belly of digastric
B. Posterior belly of digastric
C. Temporal muscle
D. Muscles of mastication
E. Mylohyoid

Ans. B

Q 59. Which of the following antibiotic acts on the bacterial walls?

    A. Clindamycin
    B. Polymyxin
    C. Ceftazidime
    D. Gentamicin
    E. Metronidazole

    Ans. C

Q 60. Which of the following is true regarding the Kleihauer test?
    A. It may be used to confirm the presence of Rhesus antibodies
    B. It should be performed routinely at 28 and 36 weeks in the woman who is rhesus negative

C. It is no longer required after delivery in the Rhesus negative woman
D. It is based on the relative resistance of foetal haemoglobin to denaturation using an acid solution
E. It is no longer required after delivery in the Rhesus negative woman

Ans. D

Q 61. Which of the following is not true regarding preimplantation genetic diagnosis?
   A. Disorders caused by a single gene defect can be detected
   B. It should be used to exclude Down syndrome in a couple undergoing IVF using a donor ovum from a 23-year-old, into a 46-year-old recipient
   C. Foetal sex can be determined
   D. HLA status can be determined
   E. It is usually not performed in natural conceptions

Ans. B

Q 62. You wish to perform karyotype analysis on a patient that you suspect has Turner's syndrome. What is the most suitable form of consent which must be obtained in this case?
   A. Consent from carer
   B. Consent from court of law
   C. Consent from next of kin if possible
   D. Verbal consent required
   E. Written consent required

Ans. D

Q 63. Which of the following structures pass under the inguinal ligament?
A. The long saphenous vein
B. The superficial femoral artery
C. The superficial epigastric vein
D. The genital branch of the genitofemoral nerve
E. The femoral branch of the genitofemoral nerve

Ans. E

Q 64. Which of the following is true concerning 1,25-(OH)$_2$ D3 (vitamin D)?
A. Facilitates calcium and phosphate reabsorption from bone
B. Is more active than 24,25-(OH)$_2$ vitamin D
C. Levels are low during lactation
D. Reduces the absorption of calcium and phosphate from the gut
E. Stimulates the excretion of calcium and phosphate into the renal tubules

Ans. B

Q 65. Which of the following is true concerning the femoral ring?
A. It is bounded laterally by the femoral artery.
B. It is bounded medially by the lacunar ligament.
C. It is lined by peritoneum.
D. It is not traversed by lymph vessels.
E. Passes deep to the inguinal ligament.

Ans. B

Q 66. Which of the following is true regarding foetal death in utero?
   A. Is usually due to diabetes
   B. Can be prevented by proper obstetric management
   C. Induction of labour should be deferred until the cervix is favourable
   D. Conception should be discouraged for at least 6 months
   E. Danazol should be prescribed to suppress lactation

Ans. B

Q 67. Which of the following is not true regarding the hormonal influence upon carbohydrate metabolism?
A. Adrenal glucocorticoids enhance the effect of glucagon
B. Catecholamines increase blood glucose concentration

C. Growth hormone increases hepatic glucose output

D. Growth hormone inhibits mobilisation of free fatty acids from adipose tissue

E. Thyroid hormones increase blood glucose concentration

Ans. D

Q 68. Which of the following is not true regarding listeria infection in pregnancy?

A. *Listeria monocytogenes* can flourish at normal refrigerator temperatures

B. It is associated with premature labour

C. It occurs in every one pregnancy out of in 1,000 in the UK

D. It is associated with eating soft cheeses, cook-chilled meals and stored foods such as coleslaw

E. This infection may be suspected if meconium is present at gestations of <34 weeks.

Ans. C

Q 69. Which of the following is true regarding Fitz-Hugh-Curtis syndrome?

A. Presents with the features of appendicitis

B. Is frequently due to tuberculosis

C. Is associated with sub-fertility

D. Is best treated by laparotomy

E. Is due to allergy to violin strings

Ans. C

Q 70. Which of the following is true regarding Bartholin's abscess?

A. Is located on the cervix uteri

B. May be associated with gonococcal infection.

C. Results from poor repair of tears sustained in childbirth.

D. Is normally treated by excision of the gland.

E. Is usually bilateral.

Ans. B

Q 71. Which of the following is true concerning genital herpes infection?
   A. Can be responsible for pre-term delivery
   B. Is always symptomatic
   C. Tender inguinal lymphadenopathy frequently occurs
   D. First attack is milder than subsequent attacks
   E. Has an incubation period of 2 months

   Ans. C

Q 72. Intrauterine infection may result in which of the following?
A. Mental handicap
B. Prematurity
C. Growth failure
D. Cerebral palsy
E. All the above

Ans. E

Q 73. Which of the following conditions is not associated with a positive Direct Coomb's test?
A. Administration of cephalosporins
B. Administration of cyclosporin
C. Haemolytic disease of the newborn
D. *Mycoplasma pneumonia*
E. Administration of methyldopa

Ans. B

Q 74. True statement regarding prostaglandins is:
A. It is synthesised from cholesterol
B. Prostaglandins are small polypeptides
C. They are secreted by the pituitary gland
D. They are secreted by the prostate gland
E. They are rarely associated with gastrointestinal side effects

Ans. D

Q 75. The incidence of a disease refers to which of the following?
- A. The number of beds occupied in a designated population with the condition
- B. The number of new cases emerging in a designated period and population
- C. The period prevalence of an illness
- D. The point prevalence of an illness
- E. The readmission rate

Ans. B

Q 76. A mother is concerned regarding her baby who has developed fractures, which appear to occur with minimal trauma. He has blue sclera. What is the most likely mode of inheritance for the baby's condition?
A. Autosomal co-dominant
B. Autosomal dominant
C. X linked recessive
D. Polygenic
E. Single gene defect

Ans. B

Q 77. In the femoral triangle, which of the following is/are true of the femoral artery?
A. Crossed by the superficial circumflex iliac vein
B. Lateral to the femoral nerve
C. Medial to the long saphenous vein
D. Posterior to the femoral branch of the genitofemoral nerve
E. Posterior to the femoral vein at the apex of the triangle

Ans. D

Q 78. Which of the following conditions should an aetiological factor satisfy before being considered to be causally related to a disease?
A. Elimination of the factor decreases the risk of the disease
B. The factor is found in all cases with the disease

C. The factor is not found among persons without the disease
D. Exposure to the factor is not required for the development of the disease
E. The factor is found more frequently among the nondiseased than the diseased

Ans. A

Q 79. Which of the following is true concerning mitochondrial DNA?
A. Is inherited from both parents
B. Is not present in spermatozoa
C. Have their own genome
D. Are scantily expressed in the neuronal tissue
E. All children of an affected mother can transmit the trait

Ans. C

Q 80. Which of the following is true regarding human immunodeficiency virus?
A. Decreases the risk of opportunistic infection
B. Induces a rise in CD4 lymphocytes, monocytes and antigen-presenting cells
C. Is a single stranded DNA retrovirus
D. Patients can be infective prior to seroconversion illness at about three months
E. The median survival with AIDS is greater than 10 years

Ans. D

Q 81. Which of the following hormones is involved with the "rescue" of the corpus luteum?
A. Prolactin
B. Chorionic gonadotropin (hCG)
C. Oestradiol
D. Oxytocin
E. Progesterone

Ans. B

Q 82. Which of the following is true regarding hypoparathyroidism?
A. May cause short stature, candidiasis and impaired nail and dental development in children
B. May be a feature of Crohn's disease
C. When due to an abnormality of the PTH receptor is termed pseudopseudohypoparathyroidism
D. Biochemically is characterised by increased calcium, increased phosphate and normal alkaline phosphatase
E. Positive Chvostek's sign can be treated with oral calcium

Ans. A

Q 83. Which of the following statement regarding endometriosis is correct?
  A. Does not usually affect the ovaries
  B. Effective drug therapy significantly improves potential fertility
  C. May be a cause of fixed retroversion of the uterus
  D. Classically causes superficial dyspareunia
  E. Tubal damage is common and occurs early in the progression of the disease

  Ans. C

Q 84. Which of the following is true regarding bacterial vaginosis?
  A. Is associated with a purulent, green discharge
  B. Is associated with pre-term labour
  C. Is associated with intense vaginitis
  D. Is associated with a cheesy smell
  E. Is best treated with tetracycline

  Ans. B

Q 85. A 33-year-old lady, who is 38 weeks pregnant, presents to her general practitioner with a 4-week history of pain and paraesthesia over the upper outer aspect of her right thigh.

There is no restriction of movements in her hips or knees and her gait is normal. Which is the most likely nerve, which is affected in this case?
A. Lateral cutaneous nerve of thigh
B. Femoral nerve
C. Common peroneal nerve
D. Sciatic nerve
E. Tibial nerve

Ans. A

Q 86. Which of the following statements is true regarding Kreb's cycle?
A. Alpha-ketoglutarate is a five-carbon molecule
B. Kreb's cycle can function under anaerobic conditions
C. Oxidative phosphorylation occurs within the cytoplasm
D. Only carbohydrates and fats are oxidised in Kreb's cycle
E. Pyruvate condenses with oxaloacetate to form citrate

Ans. A

Q 87. True regarding uric acid is:
A. Is the end-product of pyrimidine metabolism in humans
B. Is excreted mainly in the bile
C. Is highly soluble in body fluids
D. The normal blood level is 4 mg/dL
E. Its plasma levels change significantly during pregnancy

Ans. D

Q 88. Which of the following is a non-essential amino acid?
A. Arginine
B. Leucine
C. Methionine
D. Tryptophan
E. Tyrosine

Ans. E

Q 89. Raised serum iron level seen in which of the following?
A. Thalassaemia major
B. Myelodysplasia
C. Haemochromatosis
D. All the above
E. None of the above

Ans. D

Q 90. Which of the following statement regarding the effect of systemic lupus erythematosus (SLE) on the neonate is correct?
A. Neonatal SLE usually results from passively acquired maternal anti-Ro antigens
B. The most common foetal condition is congenital heart block
C. Congenital heart block occurs due to maternal autoantibodies causing reversible damage to the foetal cardiac conducting system
D. Two-thirds of surviving neonates with heart block will require a pacemaker
E. High-dose corticosteroids significantly improve foetal outcome

Ans. D

Q 91. Which of the following is not true regarding HIV infected woman?
A. Are at an increased risk of cervical dysplasia
B. Foetal transmission is more likely to occur in women with recent infection
C. Should not breast feed
D. Have no significant increase in pregnancy complications
E. Have a 50% chance of transmitting the infection to the foetus in utero

Ans. E

Q 92. A 38-years old primiparous woman with 12 weeks gestation undergoes a screening test for Down syndrome, which reveals an increased foetal risk for development of trisomy 21. Which of the following confirmatory test must be offered to her?
A. Cell-free fetal DNA sampling

B. Amniocentesis
C. Chorionic villus sampling
D. Nuchal translucency measurement
E. Cordocentesis

Ans. C

Q 93. Which of the following is not a well-recognised clinical feature of rubella infection in the first trimester?
A. Cataract
B. Hepatosplenomegaly
C. Large anterior fontanelle
D. Low birth weight
E. Purpura

Ans. C

Q 94. Which of the following is correct regarding hepatitis C in pregnancy?
A. It is most often transmitted through sexual route
B. Coexisting HIV infection increases the risk
C. Breastfeeding should be discouraged to reduce vertical transmission
D. Vertical transmission occurs in 50%
E. Caesarean section is recommended to reduce vertical transmission

Ans. B

Q 95. Which of the following is correct regarding genital herpes infection?
A. Can be responsible for pre-term delivery
B. Is always symptomatic
C. Is not caused by herpes simplex virus (HSV) type 2
D. It may be caused by herpes simplex virus type 1
E. May produce spontaneous abortion

Ans. D

Q. 96. Which of the following is/are true regarding the human

chromosomes?

A. Karyotype analysis is carried out after arresting the diving cells in anaphase stage of mitosis

B. Only the X chromosome of maternal origin is active

C. The number of Barr bodies visible at interphase in human somatic cells is always one less than the total number of X chromosomes

D. Single Barr body is found in males with Down syndrome

E. No Barr body is present in individuals with Klinefelter's syndrome

Ans. C

Q 97. Genetic counselling entails which of the following?

A. Requires chromosome culture

B. Always requires discussion of pre-natal screening

C. Involves chorionic villus biopsy

D. Involves a detailed family history

E. Usually involves marriage guidance counselling

Ans. D

Q 98. Which of the following is not correct regarding a raised MSAFP level at 16 weeks of gestation?

A. May be due to incorrect assessment of gestation.

B. May be due to gastroschisis

C. Is more likely with multiple pregnancy

D. Is more likely if the foetus has T21 (trisomy 21)

E. Is more likely after threatened miscarriage.

Ans. D

Q 99. Which of the following is true regarding a 37 year old-woman at 16 weeks' gestation?

A. Has a risk of Down syndrome of 1:100

B. Should be advised to have screening for Down syndrome

C. Should be advised to have amniocentesis, not the 'triple' test

D. Is at increased risk of Edward's syndrome

E. Is at increased risk of having a baby with a neural tube defect

Ans. D

Q 100. Attacks of hypoglycaemia are not a recognized complication of which of the following?
A. Fructosaemia
B. Galactosaemia
C. Gaucher's disease
D. Glucose-6-phosphate dehydrogenase deficiency
E. Von Gierke's disease

Ans. D

MODEL TEST PAPER 2

Time allotted: 2.5 hours

Q 1. Which of the following may reduce the anticoagulant effect of warfarin?

    A. Aspirin
    B. Oral contraceptive pills
    C. Ranitidine
    D. Diazepam
    E. Ciprofloxacin

    Ans. B

Q 2. Which of the following biochemical change typically occurs during pregnancy?
A. Increase in plasma prolactin concentration in the first trimester
B. Increase in plasma urea concentration in the second trimester
C. An increase in haematocrit in early pregnancy
D. An average reduction in tidal volume of 100 mL
E. Average 15 litres increase in total body water

Ans. A

Q 3. Which of the following regarding cellular function is not correct?
    A. Atrophy can be reversible
    B. Dysplasia can also be reversible
    C. Metaplasia is the conversion of fully differentiated cell type into another differentiated cell type
    D. Hypertrophy is the increase in cell size
    E. Neoplasia represents malignant change

    Ans. E

Q 4. Which of the following is correct regarding the diffusion of gases through the placental membrane?

A. CO_2 crosses the placenta from foetus to mother because of a high concentration gradient

B. CO_2 diffuses through the placental membrane 5 times more quickly than O_2

C. The mean PO_2 in the foetus is 50 mmHg

D. The mean PO_2 in the mother's blood is approximately 30 mmHg

E. The only way the foetus can excrete CO_2 is through the placenta

Ans. E

Q 5. Which of the following is not true regarding trophoblast?
A. Develops from the blastocyst
B. Enters the maternal circulation during normal pregnancy
C. Gives rise to the foetal blood vessels in the placenta
D. Is genetically identical to decidua
E. Replaces endothelium of pregnant spiral arterioles

Ans. D

Q 6. Which of the following term best describes the renal pathology of preeclampsia?
   A. Atheromatous plaques
   B. Glomerular hypertrophy
   C. Glomerular capillary endotheliosis
   D. Tubular vacuolization
   E. Mesangial cell hypertrophy

   Ans. C

Q 7. Hydramnios is not associated with which of the following conditions?
   A. Twin-twin transfusion syndrome
   B. Diabetes
   C. Potter's syndrome
   D. Hydrops fetalis
   E. Oesophageal atresia

   Ans. C

Q 8. Which of the following is true regarding LHRH analogues?
A. Can be used to treat endometriosis
B. Rarely cause side effects
C. Can be administered orally
D. Are inexpensive preparations
E. Act principally at the uterine level

Ans. A

Q 9. Which of the following drugs is contraindicated in the lactating woman?
A. methyl-dopa
B. Bromocriptine
C. Heparin
D. Insulin
E. Warfarin

Ans. B

Q 10. Which of the following statement regarding vitamin E is correct?
A. Is present in animal foodstuffs only
B. Its deficiency may cause intrauterine foetal death
C. It does not potentiate the action of coumarin anticoagulants
D. Is used in the treatment of infertility
E. Its dietary requirement is 10 mg per day

Ans. E

Q 11. Which of the following organelles have their own self-replicating DNA?
A. Golgi body
B. Lysosomes
C. Mitochondria
D. Nucleolus
E. Rough endoplasmic reticulum

Ans. C

Q 12. Which of the following drugs is unsafe in the last 4 weeks of pregnancy?

A. Paracetamol
B. Co-trimoxazole
C. Methylpenicillin
D. Tetracycline
E. None of the above

Ans. B

Q 13. Which of the following drug can be safely used during lactation?
A. Amantadine
B. Androgen
C. Co-amoxiclav
D. Captopril
E. None of the above

Ans. C

Q 14. Regarding drug therapy during pregnancy, which of the following statement is true?
A. Folic acid supplements are not required for the patients taking phenytoin
B. Heparin has been shown to cause central nervous system damage in the foetus if given in the second and third trimesters
C. Methyldopa is contra-indicated throughout
D. Thiazide diuretics do not reduce placental perfusion
E. Treatment with isotretinoin is a recognised indication for a termination

Ans. E

Q 15. Which of the following occurs more commonly in infants of opiate-abusing mothers?

A. Increased metabolic rate

B. Intrauterine growth retardation
C. Sudden infant death syndrome (SIDS)
D. All the above
E. None of the above

Ans. D

Q 16. Which of the following regarding metaplasia is correct?
A. Is synonymous with heteroplasia
B. In the cervix, it describes change from columnar to transitional epithelium
C. It is the change of one differentiated cell type into an undifferentiated type
D. Can be reversible
E. Represents malignant change

Ans. D

Q 17. Nalorphine can antagonise the respiratory depression caused by which of the following drugs?
A. Diazepam
B. Pentazocine
C. Pethidine
D. Thiopentone
E. None of the above

Ans. C

Q 18. Which of the following chemotherapies is/are alkylating agents?

A. Chlorambucil
B. Melphalan
C. Cisplatin
D. None of the above
E. All the above

Ans. E

Q 19. Out of the following, which is not a tocolytic agent?

A. GTN
B. Progesterone
C. Propofol
D. Salbutamol
E. Nifedipine

Ans. C

Q 20. Which of the following antibodies is secreted in large amounts in the breast milk?
A. IgA
B. IgD
C. IgE
D. IgG
E. IgM

Ans. A

Q 21. Which of the following is true regarding human chorionic gonadotropin?
A. Binds to luteinising hormone (LH) receptors
B. Has intrinsic anti-thyroid activity
C. Is a protein molecule
D. Is synthesised by the corpus luteum of pregnancy
E. Secretion peaks at 20 weeks of gestation

Ans. A

Q 22. Which of the following is true regarding the raised alphafetoprotein (AFP) levels at 16 weeks gestation?
A. Is an indication for amniocentesis
B. Is caused by gastroschisis
C. Accurate dating of pregnancy is not required for its assessment
D. May be due to Down syndrome
E. Should be confirmed by a repeat blood test

Ans. B

Q 23. Which of the following is not true regarding the routine ultrasound scan at 18– 20+6 weeks?
  A. The National Screening Committee has recommended 6 basic measurements that should be taken
  B. The National Screening Committee has identified 11 foetal anomalies to be looked for
  C. Screening for placenta praevia is at the top of the list
  D. Choroid plexus cysts no longer need any response
  E. Presence of echogenic bowel requires a response

Ans. C

Q 24. Which of the following is the possible means of diagnosis of congenital HIV infection in a neonate born to an infected mother?
A. Attempt detection of viral genome by polymerase chain reactions
B. Test for anti-p24 antibody in infant blood
C. Test for delayed hypersensitivity reactions
D. None of the above
E. All the above

Ans. A

Q 25. Which of the following micro-organisms is generally sensitive to benzylpenicillin?
A. *Streptococcus viridans*
B. *Mycoplasma pneumoniae*
C. *Cryptococcus neoformans*
D. None of the above
E. All of the above

Ans. A

Q 26. Which of the following is not true regarding cyclic AMP?
A. Activates protein kinase C
B. Activates STAT 3
C. Degraded by phosphodiesterase

D. Produced from ATP
E. Produced in response to glucagon

Ans. B

Q 27. The cyclic AMP mechanism has been shown to be an intracellular hormonal mediator for which of the following hormones?
A. Glucagon
B. Parathyroid hormone
C. Secretin
D. Vasopressin
E. All the above

Ans. E

Q 28. Which of the following is not true concerning surgical diathermy?
A. Bipolar diathermy delivers ten times more power than unipolar
B. Coagulation diathermy current has a pulsed sine wave pattern
C. Cutting diathermy current has an alternating sine wave pattern
D. Diathermy current has a frequency of 0.5 - 1 Hz
E. The current density is higher in unipolar than in bipolar diathermy

Ans. E

Q 29. At what crown-rump length would it be expected to observe the foetal heart beat using transvaginal sonography?
A. Greater than 6 mm
B. Greater than 5 mm
C. Greater than 4 mm
D. Greater than 3 mm
E. Greater than 2 mm

Ans. E

Q 30. Which of the following is not true regarding foetal pulmonary surfactant?
A. Can be detected in amniotic fluid
B. Contains more than 10% lipid
C. Contains phosphatidylglycerol
D. Is more than 40% albumin
E. Is predominantly dipalmitol phosphatidylcholine

Ans. D

Q 31. Epidural bupivacaine administered during labour may cause which of the following?
A. An increased rate of caesarean delivery
B. Decreased uterine contractility
C. Pruritus
D. Tinnitus
E. Total spinal block

Ans. D

Q 32. Which of the following is true concerning Entonox for labour analgesia?
A. Has been used since the 1990s
B. Is less effective than pethidine
C. It should be inhaled as the pains start
D. Low dose sevoflurane may be used to augment its analgesic effect
E. Should not be used with other forms of analgesia

Ans. D

Q 33. Which of the following statement regarding induction of labour is correct?
A. Can be achieved by amniotomy
B. Is easiest when the cervix is in a posterior position
C. Could be achieved by an ergometrine infusion
D. Is indicated with an uncomplicated dichorionic twin pregnancy of greater than 36 weeks' gestation
E. Cannot be achieved by intravenous prostaglandin infusion.

Ans. A

Q 34. Which of the following substances is not associated with an increased capillary permeability in cases of acute inflammation?
A. Angiotensin
B. Bradykinin
C. Histamine
D. Prostacycline
E. Serotonin

Ans. A

Q 35. Which of the following statement regarding labour is not correct?
  A. A foetal heart rate of 140 per minute is normal
  B. An acceleration in foetal heart rate after a uterine contraction is normal
  C. Braxton-Hicks contractions signify the onset of the first stage of labour
  D. Syntocinon may be given during the first and third stages of labour
  E. The placenta is delivered during the third stage

Ans. C

Q 36. Which of the following is not true regarding the normal fertilization of the human ovum?
A. Occurs in the uterus
B. Prevents further spermatozoa from entering the ovum
C. Occurs 2–5 days after ovulation
D. Occurs 5–7 days before implantation
E. Leads to the secretion of human chorionic gonadotropin within 2 weeks

Ans. A

Q 37. A team presented their audit of post-operative analgesia for pelvic surgery approximately 1 year ago from which a number of recommendations were made and changes

implemented. What is the next best step, which must be undertaken in this patient?
  A. Data analysis
  B. Re-audit
  C. Data collection
  D. Needs assessment
  E. Identification of standards

Ans. B

Q 38. Based on the recommendations by the World Health Organisation, calculation of the perinatal mortality rate (PMR) should involve which of the following?
  A. Be expressed as deaths per thousand live births
  B. Includes all deaths occurring in the first month of life
  C. Includes all foetuses and infants of gestational age of more than 20 weeks
  D. Includes all foetuses and infants weighing 500 grams or more
  E. Includes all foetuses and infants with a crown rump length of more than 35 cm

Ans. D

Q 39. Which of the following statement is correct if a characteristic is normally distributed in a population?
  A. 5% of individuals will be more than two standard deviations from the mean
  B. The mean will be greater than the median
  C. The median will be less than the mean
  D. The mode will be greater than the median
  E. The numbers of individuals above and below the mean will be equal

Ans. E

Q 40. A 40-year-old man presented with a painful swelling in the big toe and is suspected to be suffering from gout. Which blood parameter must be measured to support its diagnosis?
A. Calcium levels

B. Serum creatinine
C. Serum uric acid
D. Blood urea
E. Blood xanthine

Ans. C

Q 41. The National Screening Committee criteria for establishing a population-screening programme do not include which of the following?
  A. Clearly defined natural history of the disease
  B. Should be entirely painless
  C. There should be an effective treatment available for the condition
  D. There should be evidence that the screening test is effective at reducing morbidity or mortality
  E. Benefits of the screening test should outweigh potential harm of diagnosing and treating an asymptomatic individual picked up through screening

  Ans. B

Q 42. Which of the following describes the observation that occurs with the greatest frequency?
  A. Correlation
  B. Mean
  C. Median
  D. Mode
  E. Variance

  Ans. D

Q 43. Which of the following is not an adhesion molecule?
A. Cadherin
B. Fibronectin
C. Laminin
D. Secretin
E. Integrin

Ans. D

Q 44. Which of the following is not true concerning radiation physics?

A. A neutron has almost the same mass as a proton
B. A positron has the same size as an electron
C. A proton has a positive charge
D. An electron has a greater mass than a proton
E. The hydrogen nucleus is a proton

Ans. D

Q 45. Females differ from males in which of the following aspects?

A. Pituitary gland secretes same gonadotropic hormones in both the sexes
B. Hypothalamus shows different patterns of hormone secretion
C. Gonads do not produce gametes until later in life
D. Blood gonadotropin levels rise in later life in both the sexes
E. Polymorphs show "drumsticks" of chromatin on their nuclei

Ans. E

Q 46. Which of the following statement is correct regarding statistical distribution?

A. The mode is the value that occurs the most frequently
B. The median is that point on the scale of measurement above, which lie exactly half the values and below which lie the other half
C. Of a normally distributed variable, the probability of attaining a value higher than two standard deviations above the mean is approximately 1 in 40 (p = approximately 0.025)
D. Having a normal distribution, approximately 95% of the values will lie within the range between (mean +2 standard deviations) and (mean −2 standard deviations)
E. All the above

Ans. E

Q 47. A 26-year-old female presents with right iliac fossa pain and is taken to theatre for an appendectomy. An incision is made through the skin and onto muscle with fibres passing superiorly in an oblique direction. Into which muscle has the incision been made?
A. Transversus abdominis
B. Cremaster
C. External oblique
D. Internal oblique
E. Rectus abdominis

Ans. D

Q 48. Which of the following is true regarding Down syndrome?
A. Shows X-linked pattern of inheritance
B. There may be mild to moderate mental retardation
C. Is characterised by the presence of muscle hypertonia
D. Larger than normal space between the second and third toe
E. The commonest type of congenital heart defect, which may be present is coarctation of aorta

Ans. B

Q 49. Which of the following is not true regarding *Toxoplasma gondii*?
A. It is a cause of congenital hydrocephalus
B. It is an obligate intracellular parasite of the Apicomplexa family
C. It is identified by Gram staining
D. Is transmitted by ingestion of raw meat
E. Proliferates in the central nervous system

Ans. C

Q 50. Which of the following predispose to microbial invasion?
A. Ciliary dyskinesia
B. Cystic fibrosis
C. Neutrophil deficiency
D. All the above
E. None of the above

Ans. D

Q 51. Which of the following is suggestive of genuine stress incontinence (GSI)?
  A. Constant wetness
  B. Prolapse
  C. Dysuria
  D. Haematuria
  E. Passage of large amounts of urine

  Ans. B

Q 52. Incontinence of urine in the female is investigated by which of the following tests?
  A. Cystometry
  B. Intravenous urography
  C. Urodynamic investigations
  D. All the above
  E. None of the above

  Ans. D

Q 53. Which of the following is true regarding urge incontinence in the female?
  A. Is improved greatly by an anterior repair procedure
  B. Is improved by bladder drill and re-education
  C. Is worse during the night than at day
  D. Results in the daily passage of larger volumes of urine than normal
  E. Urodynamic studies in upper motor neuronal diseases (for example, multiple sclerosis) show an increased bladder capacity

  Ans. B

Q 54. A 25-year-old lady with 16 completed weeks of gestation has presented to the antenatal clinic with the complaints of a maculopapular rash and coryzal symptoms. Her serology

reports are as follows: Rubella IgG: positive; Rubella IgM: negative; Parvovirus B19 IgG: negative; Parvovirus B19 IgM: positive

What is the most likely diagnosis in this case?

A. Non-immunity to parvovirus B19
B. Non-immunity to rubella
C. Recent infection with rubella
D. Recent infection with parvovirus B19
E. None of the above

Ans. D

Q 55. Which of the following is a predisposing factor for the development of keloid scars?

    A. Patients of Afro-Caribbean origin with dark complexion
    B. Secondary wound closure
    C. Steroid therapy
    D. Use of local bupivacaine
    E. Triamcinolone injection

    Ans. A

Q 56. Which of the following is true regarding the vancomycin-resistant enterococci?

A. Cause resistant infective diarrhoea
B. Produce an enzyme that inactivates vancomycin
C. May be found in healthy community volunteers not recently hospitalised
D. High-dose ampicillin is the treatment of choice
E. Are commonly vancomycin-dependent

Ans. C

Q 57. Which of the following is a recognised risk associated with the use of combined oral contraceptive (COC) pills?

    A. Increased incidence of endometrial carcinoma
    B. Pelvic inflammatory disease
    C. Benign ovarian cysts
    D. Hypertension

E. Increased risk of ovarian carcinoma.

Ans. D

Q 58. Which of the following statement regarding contraception is correct?
  A. There is an increased incidence of ovarian cancer in the users of the combined oral contraceptive pill.
  B. Conversion of cholesterol to pregnenolone is the rate-limiting step in the production of sex steroid hormones.
  C. The combined oral contraceptive pill contains between 10 to 100 µg of ethinyl oestradiol.
  D. Progesterones have a major role in the treatment of threatened abortion.
  E. Contraceptive implants (e.g. Implanon) provide up to 5 years of continuous contraceptive efficacy.

Ans. B

Q 59. Presence of vaginal septa is not associated with which of the following?
A. Dysmenorrhoea
B. Dyspareunia
C. Obstructed labour
D. Uterine abnormalities
E. Easy removal in most of the cases

Ans. A

Q 60. Which of the following is true regarding Klinefelter's syndrome?
A. Is associated with hypogonadotropic hypogonadism
B. It is inherited as an X-linked disorder
C. Occurs due to non-dysjunction during mitosis
D. Is associated with severe mental retardation
E. It is associated with tall stature due to delayed fusion of the epiphysis

Ans. E

Q 61. Which of the following statement is true regarding the vagina?
A. Contains mucus-secreting glands in its epithelium.
B. During reproductive life, has an acid pH.
C. Has an anterior wall longer than the posterior wall.
D. Is derived from the mesonephric duct.
E. Is related in its lower third to the bladder base.

Ans. B

Q 62. Which of the following is true concerning the development of the genital system in a female?
A. The paramesonephric ducts develop from coelomic epithelium on the urogenital ridge
B. The sex of the embryo is determined at the 7th week of development
C. Male embryos have only the mesonephric duct whereas the female embryos have only the paramesonephric ducts
D. Mitosis in oogonia is not completed by the end of the first year of life
E. The ovary develops in the medulla of the primitive gonad

Ans. A

Q 63. Which of the following is true regarding G proteins?
A. They are involved in initiating hormone action
B. G proteins are cytoplasmic proteins
C. They are part of cell surface receptors
D. All the above
E. None of the above

Ans. D

Q 64. Which of the following is true regarding testicular feminisation syndrome?
A. Occurs due to the abnormality of the testosterone receptors
B. Is associated with 47 XXY karyotype
C. The individual is genotypically a female

D. Has undetectable serum oestrogen concentrations
E. Development of axillary/pubic hair is normal

Ans. A

Q 65. Which of the following is true regarding the fragile X syndrome?
A. Regular national screening program for fragile X syndrome exists in the UK
B. There may be small, low set ears
C. May be associated with labial/ clitoral enlargement
D. Women are more severely affected than the males
E. Women with permutation are at an increased risk of premature ovarian failure

Ans. E

Q 66. Which of the following is not true regarding the basal metabolic rate?
A. Basal metabolic rate falls with increasing age
B. Increases with increasing percent of lean body mass
C. Is greater in males than females
D. Is related to serum leptin levels
E. It is the single largest component of energy expenditure

Ans. D

Q 67. A 48-year-old woman has poorly controlled type 2 diabetes. What single test would help in determining long-term glycaemic control?
A. Fructosamine
B. Glucose
C. Glycated haemoglobin
D. Glycated albumin
E. Two hours-oral glucose tolerance test

Ans. C

Q 68. Which of the following are tumour suppressors?

A. *p53*
B. *pRb*
C. *BRCA1*
D. All the above
E. None of the above

Ans. D

Q 69. Which of the following is true regarding a baby with birthweight > 4.5 kg?
    A. Is almost always due to poorly controlled diabetes.
    B. Is not associated with an increased risk of shoulder dystocia.
    C. Is a contra-indication to vaginal delivery of a baby presenting by the breech.
    D. Another large baby is unlikely in a subsequent pregnancy.
    E. Is normally due to post-maturity.

Ans. C

Q 70. Which of the following procedures does not help correct retroversion of the uterus?
    A. Hodge pessary
    B. A laparoscopic procedure
    C. A sling operation
    D. Pelvic floor repair
    E. Gilliam's operation

Ans. D

Q 71. Which of the following is true regarding myomectomy?
    A. Is an underused alternative to hysterectomy
    B. Is useful in the management of infertility
    C. Is useful in managing menorrhagia
    D. Makes Caesarean section obligatory in subsequent pregnancy
    E. None of the above

Ans. E

Q 72. Blood supply of the vulva is derived from which of the

following?
A. Deep external pudendal artery
B. Internal pudendal artery
C. Superficial external pudendal artery
D. All the above
E. None of the above

Ans. D

Q 73. Which of the following is not true regarding the foetal circulatory system?
A. Blood flows from the foetus to the placenta in the umbilical arteries
B. The ductus arteriosus closes during labour
C. Placental circulation starts at about 1 week after implantation
D. The heart becomes a four-chamber organ at about 7 weeks' gestational age
E. Reversed end diastolic flow in the umbilical artery is associated with fetal hypoxia

Ans. B

Q 74. The lymphatic drainage of the cervix does not go to which of the following?
A. Directly to the para-aortic nodes
B. To the internal iliac nodes
C. To the obturator node
D. To the superficial inguinal nodes
E. None of the above

Ans. D

Q 75. Which of the following is true concerning gonadal development in a male?
A. Primary sex cells (gonocytes) have a haploid number of chromosomes
B. The histodifferentiation of the testis begins later than that of the ovary
C. The histological appearance of the primitive gonad is similar in

both sexes until 70 days after fertilisation
D. The paramesonephric duct totally disappears in a male
E. The interstitial cells of Leydig are derived from mesenchyme

Ans. E

Q 76. Which of the following is true regarding folic acid?
A. Bioavailability is impaired by cooking
B. Blood level is reduced in stagnant loop syndrome
C. Body stores are adequate for 3 years
D. Is absorbed predominantly in the ileum
E. It is effective treatment for alcohol-induced macrocytosis

Ans. A

Q 77. Which of the following statement is true concerning retroversion of the uterus?
A. It is a common cause of subfertility.
B. May be corrected by a Fothergill operation.
C. Should be corrected with a Hodge pessary in early pregnancy.
D. It is caused by heavyweight lifting.
E. It may occur in 20% of normal women.

Ans. E

Q 78. Which of the following is true regarding the innervation of the uterus and birth canal?
A. A paracervical nerve block may be used for a forceps delivery.
B. The pudendal nerve block provides good pain relief for the second stage of labour.
C. The parasympathetic nervous system causes contraction of the pregnant uterus.
D. The uterus contains alpha and beta receptors.
E. Pudendal nerve arises from S2 to S3 nerve roots.

Ans. D

Q 79. Which of the following is true regarding colposuspension for treatment of uterine retroversion?

A. Effectively treats dyspareunia
B. Effectively treats frequency of micuturition
C. Is an appropriate treatment for enterocoele
D. Is associated with a need to treat rectocoele
E. Is usually performed vaginally

Ans. D

Q 80. Which of the following statement is not correct regarding the mobile retroversion of the uterus?
   A. It is suspected when the cervix points anteriorly on speculum examination
   B. Is usually asymptomatic
   C. Occurs at 20 weeks gestation
   D. May occur in 20% of women
   E. Occurs in the puerperium

Ans. C

Q 81. Which of the following statement regarding thyroid gland is correct?
A. The amount of free (non-protein-bound) thyroxine (T4) in the plasma is four times less than the amount of free tri-iodothyronine (T3)
B. Thyroid hormone decreases the dissociation of oxygen from haemoglobin by increasing red cell 2,3-diphosphoglycerate (DPG)
C. Over-treatment of the pregnant mother with antithyroid drugs may result in cretinism
D. Reverse T3 is decreased in severe illness
E. Thyroid-stimulating hormone (TSH) levels are increased during normal pregnancy

Ans. C

Q 82. Which of the following is not true regarding genetic deficiency of thyroid hormone production (dyshormonogenesis)?
A. It is associated with a diminished uptake of radioactive iodine
B. Is best treated with iodine in mild cases

C. Leads to the formation of a goiter
D. May be associated with congenital nerve deafness
E. May produce no signs or symptoms of thyroid deficiency

Ans. B

Q 83. Which of the following is true regarding the ribonucleic acid?
A. Contains deoxyribose
B. It is made by RNA polymerases
C. Uracil pairs with thymine
D. It is always single-stranded
E. Adenine pairs with guanine

Ans. B

Q 84. Which of the following is true regarding cystic fibrosis?
A. It is more common amongst Caucasians
B. This disease is associated with X-linked recessive inheritance
C. The condition is due to a unique mutation
D. Pulmonary hypertension is a good prognostic feature for pregnant woman with cystic fibrosis
E. Presently neonatal screening for cystic fibrosis is not been done routinely in the UK

Ans. A

Q 85. Which of the following statement regarding dysmenorrhoea is not correct?
  A. Can be successfully treated with non-steroidal anti-inflammatory drugs
  B. Does not occur in anovulatory cycles
  C. Tends to be more severe with a retroverted uterus that is associated with a pelvic pathology
  D. Can be caused by endometriosis
  E. Can be caused by anterior vaginal wall prolapse

Ans. E

Q 86. Which of the following is correct regarding mifepristone?

A. Mifepristone has to be given parenterally

B. Mifepristone during the luteal phase effectively stops pregnancy from occurring

C. Mifepristone given in the first 7 weeks of pregnancy effectively induces abortion

D. Medical abortion with Mifepristone carries a higher risk of infection that vacuum aspiration

E. Mifepristone binds competitively to progesterone receptors and has greater affinity for them than has progesterone

Ans. E

Q 87. Which of the following correct concerning clomiphene citrate is correct?
A. It is usually started in a dosage of 100 mg daily
B. It is an antiandrogen
C. It is associated with visual disturbances
D. It produces direct induction of ovulation
E. It is usually started on day 7 of the cycle

Ans. C

Q 88. In a normal pregnancy, which of the following is true regarding uterine blood flow?
A. Is about 50 mL/minute at term
B. Is increased during uterine contractions
C. Is reduced by prostacyclin
D. Represents about 10% of the cardiac output by the end of the first trimester
E. Within the choriodecidual space is maintained throughout the cardiac cycle

Ans. E

Q 89. A 27-year-old female developed insulin dependent diabetes mellitus. Her uncle and grandmother also had diabetes mellitus. What is the most likely mode of inheritance for her condition?
A. Autosomal co-dominant
B. Autosomal dominant
C. Autosomal recessive
D. Polygenic
E. Single gene defect

Ans. D

Q 90. Which of the following vaccines must not be administered to HIV positive patients?
A. BCG
B. Havrix (hepatitis A vaccine)
C. Hib vaccine
D. Rabies virus
E. Cholera vaccine

Ans. A

Q 91. In a 20-year-old pregnant woman, acute rubella infection is diagnosed at 20 weeks of gestation. What is the most likely foetal abnormality, which is likely to occur as a result of this acute infection?
A. Cerebral palsy
B. Sensorineural hearing loss
C. Microcephaly
D. Failure to thrive
E. Limb hypoplasia

Ans. B

Q 92. Regarding the human placenta, which of the following is true?
A. Cytotrophoblast is in direct contact with maternal blood
B. Decidual cells are derived from myometrial stromal cells

C. Each cotyledon represents a primary stem villi
D. The anchoring villi are attached to the myometrium
E. The intervillous space communicates directly with branches of the uterine arteries

Ans. E

Q 93. Which of the following statement is true regarding B lymphocytes?
A. Characterised by rosette formation when mixed with sheep red cells
B. Normally the major type of circulating lymphocyte
C. The predominant cell type in the paracortical region of the lymph node
D. Produced in the lymph nodes
E. Associated with the development of humoral immunity

Ans. E

Q 94. Which of the following is true regarding fistulae due to obstructed labour?
   A. Are best repaired immediately after delivery
   B. Are commonly uretero-vaginal
   C. Are repaired by a sling operation
   D. Cause continuous urinary incontinence
   E. Are usually repaired by an abdominal approach

Ans. D

Q 95. Foetal well-being in the third trimester can be usefully assessed by which of the following parameters?
   A. Serial assessment of symphyseal fundal height
   B. Ultrasound measurement of crown–rump length
   C. Measurement of serum alpha-fetoprotein levels
   D. Measurement of serum oestradiol levels.
   E. None of the above

Ans. A

Q 96. Which of the following is not true regarding a high foetal head at term in a primipara?
    A. Can be caused by placenta praevia
    B. Can be caused by a lower-segment uterine fibroid
    C. Is associated with incorrect pregnancy dating
    D. Is an indication for a caesarean section
    E. Has a higher incidence in patients of African origin.

Ans. D

Q 97. The concentrations of which of the following increase during pregnancy?
A. Albumin
B. Sodium
C. Fibrinogen
D. All of the above
E. None of the above

Ans. C

Q 98. Which of the following is true regarding aortocaval compression in a pregnant woman?
A. A reduction in cardiac output may be due to compression of the superior vena cava
B. A wedge should be placed under the left side
C. Compression of the aorta may cause uterine hypoperfusion
D. Is greater when lying on the right side
E. Uterine contractions reduce the cardiovascular effects of aortocaval compression

Ans. C

Q 99. Which of the following is not a normal finding in a healthy pregnant patient?
A. A fourth heart sound
B. A raised alkaline phosphatase
C. Tall, peaked T waves in lead III
D. Left axis deviation on the electrocardiograph (ECG)
E. Thrombocytopenia

Ans. C

Q 100. Which of the following is true regarding the posterior pituitary gland?
A. Function is inhibited by alcohol
B. Releases decapeptide hormones
C. Secretes IGF1
D. Synthesises somatomedins
E. None of the above

Ans. A

www.ingramcontent.com/pod-product-compliance
Lightning Source LLC
Chambersburg PA
CBHW071816200526

45169CB00018B/334